Immunology
An outline for students of medicine and biology

D. M. Weir
MD, FRCPE

Reader in Immunology, Department of Bacteriology,
University of Edinburgh Medical School

FIFTH EDITION

CHURCHILL LIVINGSTONE
EDINBURGH LONDON MELBOURNE AND NEW YORK 1983

CHURCHILL LIVINGSTONE
Medical Division of Longman Group Limited

Distributed in the United States of America by
Churchill Livingstone Inc., 1560 Broadway, New York,
N.Y. 10036, and by associated companies, branches
and representatives throughout the world.

First edition   1970
Second edition   1971
Third edition   1973
Fourth edition   1977
Fifth edition   1983

ISBN 0 443 02840 0

British Library Cataloguing in Publication Data
Weir, D. M.
   Immunology. — 5th ed. — (Churchill Livingstone medical texts)
   1. Immunology
   I. Title
   616.07'9   QR181

Library of Congress Cataloging in Publication Data
Weir, D. M. (Donald Mackay)
   Immunology, an outline for students of medicine and biology.
   (Churchill Livingstone medical text)
   Includes index.
   1. Immunology. I. Title. II. Series. [DNLM:
1. Immunity. QW 504. W425i]
QR181.W392   1983   574.29   82–17839

Printed in Singapore by Selector Printing Co Pte Ltd

Preface to the Fifth Edition

Immunology continues to expand with no slackening in pace. The changes in the subject since the fourth edition of this text appeared in 1977 have necessitated a very substantial rearrangement, rewriting and updating of the material. The book is now divided into two main sections: 'Basic immunology' and 'Immunology in action'. The first section contains an outline of the basic sciences of the subject, immunochemistry and immunobiology. The second section deals with their application to the understanding of disease states including a much enlarged chapter on infection and immunity; disorders of the immune system; hypersensitivity, autoimmunity, and blood groups; transplantation and tumour immunology.

The book is written particularly for students new to the subject. There are a large number of new diagrams and tables with the emphasis throughout on simplification of difficult concepts. The lists of objectives given at the beginning of each chapter are intended to help answer the question *'How much am I expected to know?'*. The ability to achieve the objectives should provide the reader with the vocabulary used in immunology and its fundamental concepts. These serve as a background for pursuing the subject in greater depth, e.g., an honours course in immunology or related disciplines. This approach has shown itself in practice to be much appreciated by students taking course work in infection and immunity. Postgraduates requiring a revision course in immunology may find these objectives particularly useful.

I am most grateful to my wife, Dr Caroline Blackwell, for help in editing the text and for suggestions for the incorporation of new material, some of which is from our book, *Principles of infection and immunity in patient care* (Churchill Livingstone, 1981). Once again the publishers have provided invaluable editorial assistance and encouragement at all stages of the preparation.

Edinburgh, 1983 D. M. W.

Contents

Basic Immunology

1

Immunity

THE SCOPE OF IMMUNOLOGY

The tissues and cells capable of exhibiting what is now recognized as an adaptive immune response have an evolutionary history of some 400 million years and the forms taken by the response during this period have maintained a remarkable constancy both at the molecular and at the functional level. The basic pattern of the protein molecules involved has been retained, with the diversification that has occurred through evolutionary selective pressures being superimposed on this basic pattern.

Recognition

Immune phenomena as expressed in the higher animals have evolved from **recognition mechanisms** that enabled a multicellular primitive animal to distinguish between itself and other foreign species. This idea of **self–non–self discrimination** lies at the foundation of immunological theory. Self-recognition mechanisms appear very early in evolution and can be seen in marine organisms, such as sponges. Reaggregation of dispersed colonies is regulated by species-specific surface glycoproteins. Failure of adhesion of unrelated species amounts to a primitive form of graft rejection. The cells lining the cavity of sponges are able to capture microorganisms present in the water drawn into the cavity, and phagocytosis (p. 17) plays a role in the metamorphosis of insects in removing dead and disintegrated tissue.

An important recognition phenomenon occurs in the interaction between pollen grains and plant stigma, which appears to depend on the nature of surface proteins. Pollination and germination only occur if the pollen and stigma are genetically compatible and self-fertilization is prevented.

Primitive marine species such as sea stars and corals appear to be able to reject grafts of unrelated forms. Self–non-self discrimination enables the maintenance of **specific partnerships** between cells of a multicellular organism and provides an organism with the additional benefits of recognizing and excluding changed self-constituents and potentially harmful parasitic organisms, such as fungi and bacteria. The particular cell surface molecules that are recognized and determine foreignness are often carbohydrates or glycoproteins. The recognition factors themselves are proteins and it is interesting to note that the production of one of the recognition proteins (immunoglobulin M, p. 69) of the higher vertebrates is specifically stimulated by carbohydrate molecules. Immunoglobulin M is believed to represent the precursor of all the other forms of **immunoglobulin** and has its origin in the most primitive vertebrate fishes.

This had led to the view that there is a continuity between the primitive ability to recognize carbohydrates of foreign cell surfaces and the highly developed recognition factors found in higher vertebrates, which are able to discriminate between a variety of organic molecules of carbohydrate and non-carbohydrate nature.

Immunity

The meaning of the term 'immunity' as it is used today derives from its earlier usage referring to exemption from military service or paying taxes. It has long been recognized that those who recovered from epidemic diseases such as smallpox and plague were exempt from further attacks and such immune individuals were often used in an epidemic to nurse those suffering from active disease. In England the procedure of cow-pox vaccination developed by Edward Jenner in 1798 for protection against smallpox and that used by Francis Home in Edinburgh for measles protection were essentially empirical measures performed without understanding of the underlying principles.

The foundations for an understanding of immunity were laid by the invention of the microscope, the recognition of microorganisms and the advent of Pasteur's **germ theory of disease**. Pasteur's chance observation that aged cultures of chicken cholera bacillus would not cause the expected disease in chickens led to the development of methods for reducing the virulence of pathogenic microorganisms called **attenuation**. The protection given to animals by preinoculation of such attenuated organisms led to the widespread use of the method for immunization purposes.

The discovery of the tubercle bacillus by Robert Koch led him to describe the phenomenon of delayed hypersensitivity or **cell-mediated immunity** as it is known today. Immunology as a science began with the demonstration by von Behring and Kitasato at the

Koch Institute in Berlin in 1890 of an antibacterial substance or factor in the blood of animals immunized against tetanus and diphtheria organisms. The neutralizing ability of such blood serum for the bacterial toxins was the first demonstration of the effect of what is now recognized as antibody globulin.

The part played by **phagocytic cells** in clearing away and destroying bacteria was recognized by Metchnikoff, a Russian biologist working in France. Later the helpful effect of antibody (called opsonins by Almroth Wright) in encouraging phagocytosis became apparent, thus reconciling two opposing schools of thought on immune mechanisms — one believing the process to be brought about completely by blood factors and the other upholding an entirely cellular viewpoint.

Pfeiffer and Bordet demonstrated the activity of a serum factor called **complement**, which participates with antibody in the destruction of bacteria and has now been shown to have a wide variety of important biological activities. Paul Ehrlich proposed the first theory of antibody formation — **the side chain theory**. This proposed the existence of receptors on the surface of cells that could be released into the blood and neutralize bacterial toxins.

Antibody specificity
The specificity of antibody for the agent (i.e. the antigen) which induced its formation led to the use of antibody as an analytic tool. Thus the antigenic characters of bacterial and non-bacterial substances could be worked out and systems of classification of microorganisms were developed on this basis. Landsteiner used antibody-antigen interaction to define the **ABO blood group system** on the basis of antigenic differences in red cell membranes, and was also responsible for performing the ground work on the chemical basis of antigenic specificity.

Self and non-self
In more recent years, with increasing knowledge of the molecular processes underlying the functioning of cells, it became possible to formulate theories on the mechanisms whereby the tissues and cells responsible for producing antibody performed this function. The need for such theories became apparent with the recognition of human diseases where the immune mechanisms had become deranged and were treating the individual's own tissues as if they were foreign antigens. Thus the question of how the immune system distinguished between what was foreign and what was part of self became important and resulted in the formulation of new theories to ex-

plain these phenomena, notable among which was the **clonal selection** theory of Burnet. These attempted to define the scope and limitation of Ehrlich's 'contrivances by means of which the immunity reaction . . . is prevented from acting against the organism's own elements and so giving rise to autotoxin'. The advances made in this area gave a new dimension to the science of immunology which until then was devoted almost exclusively to the prevention of infectious disease by vaccination and immunization. This new field of study — **immunobiology** — has drawn the attention of biologists to the apparantly central importance of immune mechanisms in the evolution of multicellular animals.

The cells of the immune system are probably derived from the primitive cellular defence mechanism that arose with the evolution of the invertebrates. This is manifested by the engulfment and walling off of foreign particles. The phagocytic cells responsible for this do not respond by proliferation so that the animal does not become better adapted to deal more effectively with the foreign material (p. 55). It is doubtful if the immune response, as it is recognized today, first appeared with the need for protection from parasitic microorganisms but evolved in the primitive vertebrates as a way of protecting themselves from their parasitic relatives. In the absence of such protection the parasite could attach itself to a host and because the tissues of the two animals were so similar the host would be unable to react against the parasite which would thus be accepted rather like a piece of successfully grafted compatible tissue (Ch. 7). Burnet, who is one of the main exponents of this view, has suggested that the mechanism that underlies the protective response to parasites depended on the host making its own tissues antigenically different from the parasite so that the parasite could be recognized as foreign. The evolution of a defence mechanism able to resist parasitic invasion would have the added advantage of treating in the same way any tissues of the animal that changed their cell surface antigens. This, as will be discussed later (Ch. 8), is a characteristic of many tumour cells and the employment of the immunological defence mechanisms to rid the body of such cells would confer a clear evolutionary advantage to the species.

Immunity and genetics

Knowledge of the genetic control of protein synthesis is likely to make considerable advances as a result of the study of the synthesis of immunoglobulins. The concept that **two genes** may code for a **single polypeptide chain** and that groups of closely linked genes may be basic units of mammalian genomes have emerged from studies on immunoglobulin synthesis.

It is now recognized that interaction between different cell types may exert control over protein synthesis, affecting for example the particular class of immunoglobulin being manufactured by a lymphocyte (Ch. 4). The study of immunoglobulin structure has shown that in the human there are at least 10 different types and that each type contains an enormous number of variants differing slightly from each other in amino acid sequence.

The gene complex of the mouse that controls the cell surface

Table 1.1 Development of immunology

	Immunity
Late eighteenth century	Smallpox vaccination — Jenner
Late nineteenth century	Germ theory of disease, attenuated and killed vaccines — Pasteur Tubercle bacillus and cell-mediated immunity — Koch Antitoxins against diphtheria and tetanus — von Behring, Kitasato Complement activity — Pfeiffer, Bordet Agglutination of bacteria — Durham Side chain theory of immunity — Ehrlich Phagocytosis and cellular immunity — Metchnikoff

	Immunochemistry	Immunobiology
Mid-twentieth century to present day	Blood groups — Landsteiner Antigenic determinants — Landsteiner, Heidelberger, Marrack Electrophoretic separation of gamma globulin — Kabat, Tiselius Structural analysis of antibody molecule — Porter, Edelman Relationship between structure and biological activities of immunoglobulin molecule and genetic control mechanisms Determinants of immunogenicity of antigen molecule	Antiglobulin test — Coombs, Mourant, Race Recognition of autoimmunity Clonal selection theory of immunity — Burnet (Jerne) Immunological tolerance — Medawar, Owen (Glenny) Transplantation immunology, Tumour immunology, Rhesus immunization, Deficiency states, role of the thymus Immunogenetics and evolution of immune system Lymphocyte activation and products, cell cooperation Role of macrophages — antibacterial, and cytotoxic effects Monoclonal antibodies — Milstein and Kholer

antigens important in transplantation (graft) rejection has proved to be an invaluable general model for the study of the **major transplantation antigen systems** of higher vertebrates. More recently the small segment of chromosome 17 that contains this gene complex has evoked considerable interest among geneticists and immunologists. They have recognized that in addition to controlling cell surface antigens, there are closely linked genes that determine differences in level of antibody responses to many antigens, differences in susceptibility to tumour viruses and a number of other important immunological traits (Ch. 9). This gene complex is now the most thoroughly and extensively characterized segment of chromosome in any mammalian species and as such it constitutes a very valuable model for studies of gene evolution, gene action and organization.

Technical advances

Modern biochemical techniques have helped to add precision and sensitivity to immunological methods. These include the use of radioisotopes to measure accurately the primary binding of antibody with antigen and to demonstrate the metabolic activity of cells engaged in antibody production. Protein fractionation techniques and peptide analysis of the antibody molecule have thrown light on the chemical basis of specificity of the molecule and the relationship of structure to function, as well as confirming a genetic basis for antibody formation and providing factual limitations on earlier theories of antibody formation.

The understanding of immunological processes underlying the reaction of the body to tumours, to transplanted tissues and organs and to infectious agents has gained much ground as the result of these advances in immunochemical techniques. Clinical developments have included the recognition of **autoimmune** and **immunological deficiency** diseases and the feasibility of **organ transplantation**. Technical advances in the study of the in vitro behaviour of cells of the immune system and in the quantitation of serum proteins have provided valuable diagnostic help in the recognition and management of these clinical situations. Phylogenetic studies have stimulated investigations into the development and control of the lymphoid tissues leading, for example, to a new understanding of the role of that previously enigmatic organ, the thymus.

Probably the most important development in the last few years has been the emergence of techniques that come under the heading of 'genetic engineering'. The technique having a very considerable impact in many areas of the biological sciences is **monoclonal anti-**

body production, introduced by Milstein and Kholer. The method described on page 84 has led to the production of unlimited quantities of highly specific antibody to a large variety of biologically important antigens. This will revolutionize radioimmunoassay techniques (p. 235), analysis of at present ill-defined tissue and cell antigens (e.g. those of neurological tissues), treatment of tumours and auto-immunity.

The ability to introduce genetic information into bacteria and yeasts by genetic engineering techniques, leading to the production of therapeutic agents such as insulin or important viral antigens (e.g. hepatitis B antigen), is likely to have important applications over the next few years.

Thus it can be seen that immunity in its original meaning, refering to resistance to parasitic invasion by means of a specific immune response, is only one activity of a cellular system in animals. The total activity of the cellular system is concerned with mechanisms for preserving the integrity of the individual with far-reaching implications in embryology, genetics, cell biology, tumour biology and many non-infective disease processes.

The subject of immunology can be considered under three general headings: **immunity**, dealing with the adaptive response to infective agents; **immunochemistry**, concerned with the chemical nature of antigens and antibodies; and **immunobiology**, which encompasses a variety of topics of biological importance and deals with the activity of the cells of the immune system and their relationship to each other and their environment.

FURTHER READING

Brock T (ed) 1961 Milestones in microbiology. III. Immunology. Prentice-Hall, Englewood Cliffs, N.J., p 121–144
Burnet F M 1969 Changing patterns. Elsevier, New York
Foster W D 1970 A history of medical bacteriology and immunology. Heinemann, London
Good R A 1976 Runestones in immunology: inscriptions to journeys of discovery and analysis. Journal of Immunology 117: 1413
Herbert W J, Wilkinson P C 1977 A dictionary of immunology. Blackwell, Oxford
Mc Neill W H 1976 Plagues and peoples. Basil Blackwell, Oxford
Parish H J 1965 A history of immunization. Livingstone, Edinburgh

2

Innate immunity: non-specific defence mechanisms

Objectives
On completion of this section the reader will be able to:

1. Describe three host determinants of innate immunity
2. Describe with the aid of a diagram the innate immune mechanism of the skin and mucous membranes
3. Give two examples of the way that normal flora prevent infection by pathogenic microorganisms
4. Define phagocytosis and list the three essential features of the process
5. Give two examples of intracellular killing mechanisms
6. Define opsonin
7. Describe in outline the differences between complement activation by the classical and alternate pathways; give three examples of the biological activities of complement activation products
8. Describe the three main features of an inflammatory response and give two examples of endogenous mediators of inflammation

The healthy individual is able to protect himself from potentially harmful microorganisms in the environment by a number of very effective mechanisms, present from birth, which do not depend upon having previous experience of any particular microorganism. The innate immune mechanisms are **non-specific** in the sense that they are effective against a wide range of potentially infective agents. The main determinants of innate immunity seem genetically controlled, varying widely with species and strain and to a lesser extent between individuals. Age, sex and hormone balance play lesser roles. In comparison, acquired immune mechanisms, discussed below, depend upon the development of an immune response to individual microorganisms that is specific only for the inducing organism.

Determinants of innate immunity

Species and strain

Marked differences exist in the susceptibility of different species to infective agents. The rat is strikingly insusceptible to diphtheria whilst the guinea-pig and man are highly susceptible. The rabbit is particularly susceptible to myxomatosis and man to syphilis, leprosy and meningococcal meningitis. Susceptibility to an infection does not always imply a lack of resistance because, although man is highly susceptible for the common cold, he overcomes the infection within a few days. Dogs in contrast are not susceptible to the virus agents responsible for the common cold in man. In some diseases, although a species may be difficult to infect (i.e. insusceptible), once established the disease can progress rapidly (i.e. lack of resistance). For example rabies, although common to both man and dogs, is not readily established as the virus does not easily penetrate healthy skin. Once infection is established, however, the resistance mechanisms in both species are not able to overcome the disease. Marked variations in resistance to infection between different strains of mice have been noted.

Table 2.1 Determinants of innate immunity

Specific host determinants	Physical determinants	Active anti-microbial determinants
Species and strain	Skin and mucous membrane barriers, moist surfaces	Antibacterial and antifungal secretions of skin — sweat and sebaceous secretions
Individual genetic factors	Anatomical traps, e.g. nasal cavity	Antibacterial and antiviral secretions of mucous membranes
Age	Mechanical cleansing, e.g. cilia	Antimicrobial substances of tissue fluids, e.g. lysozyme, basic polypeptides Phagocytosis and digestion
Hormonal balance		

In man the habits and environment of a community affect his ability to resist particular infections by acquired immune mechanisms developing early in life. This environmentally determined type of resistance is easily confused with the genetically controlled innate immunity and makes it difficult to ascertain differences in innate immunity in different communities. It is, however, fairly clear that the American Indian and the Negro are more susceptible to tuberculosis than are Caucasians. It seems reasonable to assume that certain interspecies and interstrain differences have arisen by a process of natural selection.

Individual differences and influence of age
The role of heredity in determining resistance to infection is well illustrated by studies on tuberculosis infection in twins. If one homozygous twin develops tuberculosis, the other twin has a three to one chance of developing the disease compared to a one in three chance if the twins are heterozygous. Sometimes genetically controlled abnormalities are an advantage to the individual in resisting infection, as for example in a hereditary abnormality of the red blood cells (sickling) which are less readily parasitized by *Plasmodium falciparum*, thus conferring insusceptibility to malaria. Infectious diseases are more severe at the extremes of life, and in the young animal this appears to be associated with immaturity of the immunological mechanisms affecting the ability of the lymphoid system to deal with and react to foreign antigens. In the elderly, on the other hand, physical abnormalities (e.g. prostatic enlargement leading to stasis of urine) are a common cause of increased susceptibility to infection.

Nutritional factors and hormonal influences
The adverse effect of poor nutrition on susceptibility to infectious agents is usually not seriously questioned. Experimental evidence in animals has shown repeatedly that inadequate diet may be correlated with increased susceptibility to a variety of bacterial diseases and this has been associated with decreased phagocytic activity and leucopenia. In the case of infective agents such as viruses, which depend upon the normal metabolic function of the host cells, malnutrition, if it interfered with such activities, would be expected to hinder proliferation of the potentially infective agent. There is experimental evidence in support of this view in a number of animal species, which when undernourished were less susceptible to a variety of viruses including vaccinia virus and certain neurotropic viruses. The same may be true of malaria infections in man. The parasite requires para-amino benzoic acid for multiplication and this may be deficient when a low level of nutrition exists. The exact role of nutritional factors in resistance to infectious agents in man is difficult to determine by epidemiological data. Poor diet is often associated with poor environmental conditions and increased incidence of infection can correlate with poor sanitary conditions.

There is decreased resistance to infection in diseases such as diabetes mellitus, hypothyroidism and adrenal dysfunction. The reasons for this have yet to be elucidated in detail, but, in the case of adrenal dysfunction, it is known that the glucocorticoids are anti-inflammatory agents, decreasing the ability of phagocytes to digest ingested material (probably by stabilizing the lysozomal membranes).

Mechanisms of innate immunity

Mechanical barriers and surface secretions

The intact skin and mucous membranes of the body afford effective protection against non-pathogenic organisms and a high degree of protection against pathogens (Fig. 2.1 and Table 2.2). The skin is the more resistant barrier because of its outer horny layer. The damp surface of the mucous membranes of the respiratory tract acts as a trapping mechanism and, together with the action of the hair-like processes or cilia, sweeps away foreign particulate material so that it passes into the saliva and then is swallowed. Various physi-

SKIN

Antifungal and antibacterial sebaceous secretions and sweat	SECRETIONS
Strateum corneum	MECHANICAL BARRIER
Sebaceous gland	
Phagocytic cells	INITIATES ACQUIRED IMMUNITY
Hair follicle	
Sweat gland	
Antibacterial substances in tissue fluid	

RESPIRATORY MUCOUS MEMBRANE

Moist surface bactericidal and viricidal secretions	SECRETIONS
Cilia	MECHANICAL BARRIER
Epithelium	
Muscle layer	
Gland	
Phagocytic cells	INITIATES ACQUIRED IMMUNITY
Antibacterial substances in tissue fluid	

Fig. 2.1 Innate immune mechanisms

Table 2.2   Resistance to infection: surface defences

Skin
— horny layer (*stratum corneum*) mechanical barrier
— desquamation; loss of superficial layer with attached microorganisms
— skin microflora; e.g. *Proprionobacterium acnes* produces antibacterial fatty acids
— sweat and sebaceous secretions, lactic acid and fatty acids lower pH of skin, lysozyme of sweat kills Gram +ve bacteria

Mucous membranes
— epithelial layer with damp mucous surface attaches bacteria
— cilia of respiratory tracts and coughing sweeps out foreign particles
— normal flora prevent colonization of gut by foreign organisms, degrade biliary acids, use up essential nutrient
— lysozyme in saliva kills Gram +ve bacteria
— acid production by lactobacilli in vagina — antibacterial
— flow rate of fluids over mucous membranes, e.g. keeps urinary tract sterile
— antibacterial substances secreted in mucous secretions, e.g. lysozyme, complement, interferon, transferin, lactoferin, virus inhibiting glycoproteins
— Phagocytic cells, polymorphs and macrophages
Components of the immune system, e.g. lgA, lgG, lgM, lymphocytes and macrophages

Defences of tissues
— serum components, antibacterial factors, e.g. complement, lysozyme, lactoferin, transferin, β-lysin, interferon, glycoproteins
— Phagocytic cells
— Components of the immune system. Humoral and cell-mediated immunity

General influences
— Nutritional, endocrine and metabolic factors
— Age and genetic factors

cal, chemical and microbiological agents can be toxic to cilia. Respiratory viruses, particularly influenza, and pathogenic *Mycoplasma pneumoniae* interfere with ciliary activity.

There are no cilia in the gastrointestinal tract but the layer of mucus can trap organisms and the effect of peristalsis prevents bacterial overgrowth. Slowing of normal intestinal mobility is likely to lead to increased numbers of gut bacteria and, if the mucosal barrier is damaged, leakage of microorganisms can occur with potentially serious results.

On reaching the stomach the acid gastric juices destroy any microorganisms present. Nasal secretions and saliva contain mucopolysaccharides capable of inactivating some viruses and the tears contain lysozyme active against Gram-positive bacteria. The sebaceous secretions and sweat of the skin contain bactericidal and fungicidal fatty acids and these constitute a very effective protective mechanism against potentially pathogenic microorganisms. The antimicrobial substances include the sweat gland secretions: lactic acid, amino acids, uric acid, and ammonia (the acidity of sweat, pH 5.5, has a microbicidal effect); the sebaceous secretions: triglycerides, free fatty acids and wax alcohols; substances derived from the cornification process: steroids, amino acids, pentoses, phospholipids, and complex polypeptides. Certain areas of the body such as the soles of the feet are deficient in sebaceous glands and this explains in part why such areas are susceptible to fungal infection. These are sometimes referred to as alkaline gaps. The protective ability of these secretions varies at different stages of life and it is known that fungal 'ringworm' infection of children disappears at puberty.

Areas where there is a high flow rate of secretions such as the urinary tract, biliary tract and lower respiratory tract are generally sterile in contrast to areas where the flow rate is slower, such as the oropharynx and the large bowel. Interference with flow rate in the urinary tract or biliary tract will lead to infection.

Bactericidal substances of the tissues and body fluids

Lysozyme. This is a low molecular weight basic protein found in relatively high concentration in polymorphonuclear leucocytes as well in most tissue fluids except CSF, sweat and urine. It functions as a mucolytic enzyme, splitting sugars off the glycopeptides of the cell wall of many Gram-positive bacteria, resulting in their lysis. Lysozyme may also play a role in the intracellular destruction of some Gram-negative bacteria. This antibacterial agent was described by Fleming who in 1922 was able to measure its effect on a particular Gram-positive organism, *Micrococcus lysodeikticus.* Human tears contain a large quantity of lysozyme and egg white is a rich commercial source.

Lysozyme is synthesized in the parotid gland, in the mucosa of the respiratory and gastrointestinal tracts and in the spleen and lymph nodes. Mononuclear phagocytes make lysozyme and polymorphonuclear granulocytes contain lysozyme but do not synthesize it. Thus protection by lysozyme is brought about by its local synthesis and release into the mucous secretions and by mononuclear phagocytes that infiltrate a tissue during an inflammatory response and release it at that site. The release of lysozyme from the breakdown of granulocytes has the same effect. The importance of lysozyme in phagocytic cells in protection from pathogenic microorganisms is indicated by a reported defect in bacterial killing by leucocytes from a person in whom lack of lysozyme was demonstrated. The possibility has been suggested, on the basis of in vitro work with tumour cells exposed to lysozyme, that lysozyme secreted locally by macrophages may play a role in the prevention of tumour growth. Macrophages are known to be a prominent cell in the inflammatory response associated with tumours.

Basic polypeptides. A variety of basic proteins, derived from the tissue and blood cells damaged in the course of infection and inflammation, have been found in the tissues of animals. This group includes spermine and spermidine, which kill tubercle bacilli and some staphylococci, and the arginine- and lysine-containing basic proteins protamine and histone. The ability of these basic polypeptides to destroy bacteria probably depends on the ability of the NH_2 groups to react non-specifically with the nearest acidic substance.

Humoral factors and phagocytes

A number of other so-called 'acute phase' materials are present in the blood and increase in level in the inflammatory response: C-reactive protein, $\alpha 1$ antitrypsin, $\alpha 2$ macroglobulin, fibrinogen, and caeruloplasmin, and certain complement components. The increase in level of these proteins appears to be mediated by a protein termed leucocytic endogenous mediator that is released by phagocytes. The role of many of these acute phase substances is not clear, but C-reactive protein and microorganisms can activate complement by the classical pathway. There is also evidence that C-reactive protein can bind to both human and mouse T lymphocytes, resulting in the reduction of their activity in certain immune functions. In such a situation, interference with normal immune mechanisms would be expected. Some of the other acute phase substances may also interfere with immunoregulatory mechanisms, and as indicated in Chapter 5, may account for some aspects of the immunosuppression noted in various infections (see Table 5.2).

Normal bacterial flora and protection from infection

The normal bacterial flora of the skin may itself produce various antimicrobial substances such as bacteriocins, and acids. At the same time the normal flora compete with potential pathogens for essential nutrients.

There are a very large number of microorganisms that live in close association with man — around 10^{12} bacteria on the skin and about 10^{14} in the gut (see p. 109, Figs 5.1–3). Probably the most valuable function these 'commensal' organisms serve is the exclusion of other microorganisms. Other functions include the degradation of bile acids as well as providing stimulation of the immune system to microbial antigens. The latter role is illustrated by the observation that germ-free animals make only about 1/50th as much immunoglobulin as conventional animals. If the commensal organisms of the gut are removed by antibiotics, pathogenic organisms can readily gain a foothold. Experiments with mice have shown after sterilisation of the gut with streptomycin the animals can be killed with 1/10 000 the dose of *Salmonella typhimurium* required to kill the untreated animals. Guinea pigs given penicillin undergo a profound change in the microbial content of the bowel. Such organisms may then get into the bloodstream and kill the animal. The lactobacilli of the vagina ferment glycogen and reduce the pH to about 4. If this flora is disturbed by antibiotics, other bacteria, yeasts or parasites can become established.

These observations point to the importance of not disturbing the relationship between host and its indigenous flora. Damage to the respiratory mucosa, for example by smoking, is likely to be followed by alteration in the normal flora and replacement by pathogenic organisms. Commensal organisms from the gut can cause infection in an area that they do not normally populate. An example of this is urinary tract infections resulting from the introduction of *E. coli* by means of a urinary catheter. These commensals that are given the circumstances in which to cause infections are called 'opportunistic pathogens'. Infections with these opportunists are quite widespread, often appearing as a result of medical or surgical treatment (see the compromised host, p. 108).

Phagocytosis and the inflammatory response
Microorganisms or inert particles such as colloidal carbon entering the tissue fluids or bloodstream are very rapidly engulfed by various circulating and tissue-fixed phagocytic cells. These cells are of two types, the **polymorphonuclear** leucocytes of the blood — or microphages as they are sometimes called — and the **mononuclear** phagocytic cells distributed throughout the body, both **circulating** in the blood and **fixed** in the tissues. The latter cells make up the cells of the reticuloendothelial system or RES and are given the generic name macrophages. Macrophages in the blood are known as monocytes, those in the connective tissues as histiocytes, those in the spleen, lymph nodes and thymus as the sinus-lining macrophages (sometimes called reticulum cells).

It is now established that the macrophages of connective tissues are derived from the peripheral blood monocytes as are the Kupffer cells of the liver, the alveolar macrophages of the lungs, and the free macrophages of the spleen, lymph nodes and bone marrow. In the spleen and lymph nodes, both free and fixed macrophages occur in close association with the reticular cells, which act as a framework for the macrophages. The reticular cells themselves, although able to ingest particulate material, are not regarded as mononuclear phagocytes, nor are the dendritic cells (p. 52) of the follicles of the spleen and lymph nodes. The term **mononuclear phagocyte system** describing actively phagocytic cells is now widely accepted as more satisfactory description of the function, origin and morphology of phagocytes than the older RES classification, which included actively and poorly phagocytic cells.

The three essential features of these phagocytic cells are (1) that they are actively **phagocytic**, (2) that they contain **digestive enzymes** to degrade ingested material and (3) that the macrophages are an important **link** between the innate and the acquired immune mechanisms, partly by passing on antigens or their products to the lymphoid cells and partly by retaining antigens to ensure that lymphoid cells are not overwhelmed by excess antigen (p. 60).

The process of phagocytosis is undoubtedly one of the earliest accomplishments of living cells. At the beginning of the century Metchnikoff in Russia first appreciated the continuity of this function through evolution and the important role of this activity in resistance to infectious agents.

The role of the phagocyte in innate immunity is to engulf particulate (phagocytosis) or soluble material (pinocytosis) and either to digest it or if indigestible to store it away so that it no longer serves as a local irritant, e.g. carbon particles from a polluted atmosphere.

The macrophages of the mononuclear phagocyte system serve a very important role in clearing the bloodstream of foreign particulate material such as bacteria. The efficiency of this process can be dramatically illustrated by injecting colloidal carbon into the circulation of a mouse. Samples of blood taken at short intervals thereafter show a very rapid removal of most of the particles within a few minutes after injection and the blood is completely cleared by 15 to 20 minutes. Dissection of the animal will show massive localisation of the carbon particles, particularly in Kupffer cells of the liver, of the spleen sinus-lining macrophages and in the macrophages of the lungs. This system of phagocytic cells has an enormous capacity to take up material from the blood and the finding of free microorganisms in the bloodstream usually means that there is a continued release of organisms from an abscess or from the bacterial 'vegetation' found in bacterial endocarditis.

There are many examples of the ability of the phagocytic cells of animals to ingest and dispose of different kinds of microorganisms. The destruction of phagocytic cells by chemical agents in the rabbit results in the animal losing resistance to a normally avirulent pneumococcus. The enhanced ability of macrophages from animals infected with tubercle bacilli or listeria to resist these and other infective agents is discussed on page 121. Some microorganisms such as brucellae and streptococci can resist intracellular digestion (p. 113).

The way in which phagocytes **recognize, bind** and **ingest** particulate materials such as microorganisms is only beginning to be understood. Initial adherence depends on two distinct mechanisms.

1. Relatively non-specific binding that appears to depend, as shown by work in the author's laboratory, on cell surface glycoproteins of the phagocyte binding to cell wall carbohydrates of the microorganism. This ability is probably derived from the recognition abilities found in primitive species discussed in Chapter 1 and has been retained during evolution.

2. More recently evolved mechanisms that utilize receptors in the phagocyte cell membrane for a part of the antibody molecule (Fc component, p. 72) and for a component of the complement system (C3b, p. 23). Microorganisms coated with antibody and complement thus adhere to the phagocyte and can then be ingested. Antibodies can markedly enhance the activities of phagocytic cells and even improve intracellular digestion. Such antibodies are known as **opsonins** (p. 73).

Injury to tissue excites an inflammatory response. Three major changes are associated with the inflammatory response to invading microorganisms:

1. changes in vascular calibre and blood flow
2. increased permeability in the walls of arterioles, capillaries and venules leading to fluid exudation and swelling
3. passage of leucocytes through the blood vessel walls via the interendothelial junctions into the surrounding tissues (diapedesis).

These changes are brought about mainly by chemical mediators with a minor role played by nerve impulses. There are two types of mediator, exogenous and endogenous. Bacterial products can act as exogenous mediators and can be directly responsible for increased vascular permeability and leakage of fluid and leucocytes. Such products can also attract leucocytes to the site of infection by a process known as chemotaxis. Endogenous mediators are of more importance in inflammation and can be classified into two major groups — those from the blood and those from the tissues (Table 2.3).

Table 2.3   Endogenous mediators of inflammation

Blood fluids:	Complement components (C_3 and C_5 fragments
	  — anaphylatoxins
	  — chemotaxins
	Components of clotting system
	  — Fibrinopeptides
	  — Fibrin
	  degradation products
	Kinin system
	  — Hageman factor
	  — Kallikrein
	  — Bradykinin
		vascular permeability changes, attraction of leucocytes, activation of leucocytes, contraction of smooth muscle, dilatation of blood vessels, pain and swelling

Tissues and cells:	Vasoactive amines
	  — histamine
	  — 5-hydroxytryptamine
	  — prostaglandins and
	  acidic lipids
	Lysosomal enzymes
	Non-antibody lymphocyte products
	  — MIF chemotactic
	  factors etc.	

Antimicrobial activities of phagocytes

Phagocytes, as noted above, can bind microorganisms by various membrane receptors. The organism is phagocytosed and taken into a phagocytic vacuole (a phagosome) that then fuses with an enzyme-containing lysosomal granule. The formation of this phago-lysosome usually results in the destruction of the microorganism. There are two main systems involved: the oxygen-dependent one and the oxygen-independent one, the former being the most powerful. In the **oxygen-dependent system** (the peroxidase-myeloperoxidase-halide system), phagocytosis is followed by an increase in hexose monophosphate shunt activity. This leads to conversion of oxygen to superoxide anion, hydrogen peroxide, singlet oxygen and hydroxyl radicals. These are all able to destroy microorganisms. Myeloperoxidase generates free halide ions that have powerful bactericidal and viricidal activities. The **oxygen-independent agents** include low pH, lysozyme, lactoferrin, leukin, phagocytin and a variety of hydrolytic enzymes that damage bacterial cell walls and result in digestion of the microbe.

In general, neutrophils generate more toxic oxygen components than monocytes and macrophages and are more effective at rapid killing of microorganisms. Macrophages are more versatile than the polymorphs and are crucial to the elimination of a variety of chronic infective agents as well as participating in a number of immuno-regulatory processes.

Many successfully infective microorganisms resist killing and digestion in phagocytic vacuoles and certain organisms are adapted to growing in phagocytes. Specific examples will be found in Chapter 5.

Phagocytin. Extracts of the cytoplasm of polymorphonuclear leucocytes from several species have been found to contain an acid-soluble protein bactericidal for Gram-negative bacteria and also for a few Gram-positive organisms. Phagocytin is present together with other antibacterial substances in the granules of polymorphs.

Temperature

The temperature dependence of many microorganisms is well known and tubercle bacilli, pathogenic for mammalian species, will not infect cold-blooded animals. Hens, which are naturally immune to anthrax, can be infected if their temperature is lowered. Gonococci are readily killed at temperatures over 40°C and fever therapy was a common treatment of gonococcal infection before the introduction of antibiotics.

It is therefore apparent that temperature is an important factor in determining the innate immunity of an animal to some infective agents and it seems likely that the **pyrexia** which follows so many different types of infection can function as a **protective** response against the infecting microorganisms. Recent evidence shows that human lymphocytes cultured at 39° and 41°C show enhanced responsiveness to plant haemagglutinins (p. 92) and streptococcal products.

The complement system

The existence of a heat-labile serum component with the ability to lyse red blood cells and destroy Gram-negative bacteria has been known for the last 50 years or so. The chemical complexity of the phenomenon was not initially appreciated by early workers who ascribed the activity to a single component — **complement**. Complement is an extremely complex group of serum proteins, present in low concentration in normal serum, consistently of at least 17 different proteins. Because of its broad range of biological effects, complement activation has been implicated in a variety of physiological situations. Complement activation may be linked to other humoral mediators of inflammation including the kinin and clotting systems. In model systems, one of the components, C3, seems to play a role in the development of immunological memory (p. 86) and the switch from IgM to IgG in the primary immune response (p. 83) to certain types of an antigen.

Complement components have the characteristic of interacting with certain antibody molecules once these have combined with antigen. These components are best known for their ability to combine with anti-erythrocyte antibody attached to the red cell membrane, the effect of complement being to bring about lysis of the red cell by what appears to be enzymic digestion of small areas of the cell membrane. Much of what is known today about the complement system comes from studies of immune haemolysis.

Complement, together with the blood clotting, fibrinolytic and kinin generating systems, are triggered enzyme cascade systems. The first three complement components, C1,4 and 3, circulate in an inactive form as proenzymes and are converted to their active form by their predecessors in the cascade. Complement components are not all synthesized by a single type of cell and are all fairly large proteins, C3 being the most abundant with a concentration of about 1200 μg/ml serum. The intestinal epithelium, macrophage, liver and spleen are the main sources of the components.

It is now established that the system can be activated in two different ways, the classical pathway and the alternate pathway. The events proceed in a sequential fashion by conformational changes in a protein complex by breaking peptide bonds to release fragments of the original molecule. These fragments are given small letters, the major fragments being assigned the letter b, e.g. C3b, and the smaller peptides usually given an a, e.g. C3a. In both the classical and alternate pathways C3 activation is the common central event. The **classical pathway** is typically initiated by complexes of antibody and antigen in solution or on the surface of a cell. IgM, IgG$_1$, IgG$_2$ and IgG$_3$ subclasses in particular are complement-activating, whereas IgG$_4$, IgA, IgD and IgE are not (p. 72).

An outstanding feature of the activation of the classical complement pathway is the fragmentation or cleaving of individual components into **large** fragments, which enter into combination with other complement components, and **small** fragments, which have other biological activities described later.

There are three separate stages involved in the activation of the complement system, the recognition stage, the activation stage, and the membrane attack stage. It is usual in the complement literature to show a bar over the complement enzymes and activated components formed during the activation process, e.g. C$\overline{567}$, but this has been avoided here for simplicity.

1. The **recognition stage** involves an interaction between the first component of complement C1 (the recognition unit) and a complement binding site on an immunoglobulin molecule. The complement binding site is not available on the native Ig molecule and becomes exposed after conformational changes in the molecule following interaction with antigen. The complement binding site is present in the Fc fragment of the immunoglobulin molecule (see p. 72) and in the IgM molecule has been found to be associated with a particular part of the Fc fragment called the CH_3 domain (p. 68).

The C1 component is made up of three distinct proteins held together by calcium ions, C1q, C1r and C1s. C1q is the recognition protein and binds to the exposed site on the Fc fragment of the immunoglobulin molecule. It is believed that C1q binding induces conformational changes in the C1 complex resulting in conversion of C1r to an enzyme capable of activating C1s.

2. The **activation stage** in which activated C1s acts on C2 and C4 components results in the production of a C2, C4 complex known as C3 convertase. This enzyme then acts on C3 and splits C3 into a small and a large subunit, C3a and C3b. C3a is released into the body fluids. C3b in association with its activating enzyme forms another enzyme, C5 convertase, and this leads on to the last stage.

3. The **membrane attack** stage. This occurs when the recognition and activation stages have taken place on the surface of a cell such as an erythrocyte, used in in vitro serological tests with complement, or on a bacterium invading the tissues. This membrane attack sequence is initiated by the reaction of C5 convertase on the next complement component C5. Once again a small fragment C5a is split off and released into the body fluids. A larger C5b fragment remains bound to the activating complex. This leads to the incorporation of the remaining complement components C6–9 without further enzymic action and consequent lysis of the red cell or bacterium. The biochemical events associated with the interaction of these later components with the C1425 complex are not understood but are thought to be due to an effect on a phospholipid component of the cell membrane. The result is the production of nearly circular holes $0.8-1.0$ μm in diameter in the red cell membrane and loss of its contents (Fig. 2.2).

The **alternate** or **by-pass** pathway misses out the C1, C4 and C2 components and starts at the C3 step. The components C3–C9 are depleted when this pathway is activated although for some unknown reason the system is poorly lytic. This alternate pathway is independent of the Fc portion and can be initiated by aggregated immunoglobulin (IgG, IgA and possibly IgE) or F(ab)₂ fragments (see p. 65) and also by various polysaccharides including endotoxin, zymosan and agar. These substances, in the presence of magnesium ions, convert factor B (formerly C3 proactivator) into C3 activator, which splits C3 into the small C3a subunit and the large C3b subunit. Activation of the alternate pathway in the absence of antibody yields the same biologically active products as the classical pathway. These products help in the first-line host defence against microorganisms and mediate inflammatory changes in the absence of antibody.

Uncontrolled activation of the complement system is avoided in part by the lability of the activated components and by several serum proteins that limit activation. These include a C1 esterase inhibitor and the important controlling protein C3b inactivator that cleaves C3b into at least two fragments, as shown in Figure 2.2.

Red cell lysis, whilst the most intensively studied complement activity, is by no means the only role played by the complex. Complement action is of some considerable importance because of its ability to neutralise various types of cell such as human cells or Gram-negative bacteria after they have interacted with antibody. Complement appears to render the bacteria susceptible to lysozyme. Tumour cells for example can survive indefinitely in the presence of antibody but on the addition of complement the cells develop blebs in the membrane, become fragile and lose many of

Fig. 2.2 Simplified view of activation of complement pathways and activities of components

their intracellular constituents, leading to death of the cell. Another extremely important role of complement is in the attraction of poly-morphonuclear phagocytes to sites of antigen-antibody interaction. This important step in the inflammatory process is known as **chemotaxis** and appears to depend on the components C5, 6 and 7 interacting with the C1, 4, 2, 3 complex. C5a itself has a chemotactic effect. In hypersensitivity states (Ch. 9) complement activation is responsible for the formation of substances known as **anaphylatoxins** three of which are identifiable by MW differences (7500, 8500 and 10 000). They arise after C3 and C5 activation and are responsible for bringing about the release of histamine leading to increased vascular permeability and smooth muscle contraction. The formation of the plasma kinins, e.g. C-kinin, which are active in hypersensitivity states, also appears to depend upon complement activation. Complement components C1–C3 are concerned in promoting phagocytosis and act as **opsonins** (p. 73). Table 2.4 shows some of the biological effects of activation products of the complement system.

Table 2.4   Biological effects of activation products of complement system

Complexes and components involved	Activities
C1,4	Neutralization of herpes simplex virus together with IgM
C1,4,2	Possible generation of kinins, increase in vascular permeability
C3b	Immune adherence, C3b on rbc[1], wbc[2] or platelet adheres to normal rbcs — agglutination in vitro Viruses coated with Ig and complement adhere to platelets or rbcs resulting in removal by phagocytes
C3a	Anaphylatoxin (contraction of smooth muscle, increased vascular permeability and histamine release)
C3e[3]	Mobilization of leucocytes (leucocyte promoting factor)
C3b, C5a	Stimulation of oxidative metabolism of phagocytes
C5a	Leucocyte chemotaxis Anaphylatoxin Adherence of leucocytes to vascular endothelium
C5–9	Lysis of susceptible bacteria or cells
C8, 9	Cytotoxic effect

[1] red blood cell
[2] white blood cell
[3] C3e appears to be derived from C3c by proteolytic cleavage which is itself derived from C3b by the action of β1H globulin and the C3b inactivator.

Many cells of the lymphoid system have receptors for complement components. Macrophages and B lymphocytes (p. 77), for example, react with split products of C3 (C3b), which may play a part in triggering the activation of the lymphocyte and in phagocytosis by macrophages of antigen-antibody complexes with bound complement.

Normal human serum, as noted above contains an inhibitor (an α_2-neuraminoglycoprotein) of C1 esterase. This inhibitor may be quantitatively or qualitatively deficient and lead to the condition known as hereditary angioneurotic oedema. The effects are probably due to the formation of anaphylatoxins with the consequent release of histamine. Complement deficiencies are rare, but hereditary deficiencies of the C1 components, C2 and C4 are accompanied in many cases by a variety of chronic diseases, including recurrent infections and renal disease. In laboratory practice complement lysis tests have wide and important applications (p. 239).

FURTHER READING

Austen K F 1974 The immunobiology of complement. Transplant Proceedings 6:1
Bacteriological Reviews 1960 Symposium on mechanisms of non-specific resistance
    to infection. Bacteriological Reviews 24:1
van Furth R 1975 Mononuclear phagocytes in immunity. Blackwell, Oxford
Howard J G 1963 Natural immunity. In: Cruickshank R (ed) Modern trends in
    immunology, I. Butterworth, London
Lachmann P J, Peters D K 1982 Clinical aspects of immunology, 4th edn. Blackwell, Oxford.
Mackaness G B, Blanden R V 1967 Cellular immunity. Progress in Allergy 11: 89
Müller-Eberhard H J 1975 Complement. Annual Review of Biochemistry 44: 697
Nelson D S 1976 Immunobiology of the macrophage. Academic Press, New York
Schur P H, Austen K F 1968 Complement in human disease. Annual Review of
    Medicine 19:1
Vogt W 1974 Activation, activities and pharmacologically active products of
    complement. Pharmacological Reviews 28: 125

3

Antigens

Objectives

One completion of this section the reader will be able to:
1. Define immunogen and hapten
2. Describe the concept of 'foreign' in terms of the immune system
3. List three important determinants of antigenic specificity
4. List three molecular requirements for immunogenicity.

Antigens are substances of various chemical types capable of stimulating the immune system of an animal to produce a response specifically directed at the inducing substance and not other unrelated substances. The specificity of the immune response for chemical structures (antigenic determinants) of the antigen molecule is an important characteristic. An antibody directed against an antigenic determinant of a particular molecule will react only with this determinant or another **very similar** structure. Even minor chemical changes in the determinant with the resulting change in shape will markedly alter the ability of the determinant to react with antibody. The term antigen, referring to substances capable of acting as specific stimulants of the immune response or reacting with antibody in an in vitro serological test, is used rather loosely by immunologists.

Immunogens and haptens

Substances which de novo are capable themselves of inducing an immune response are sometimes referred to as **immunogens** and are usually large molecules. In contrast, substances (often simple chemicals) incapable alone of inducing an immune response are termed **haptens**. To induce an immune response the hapten requires to be attached to a carrier molecule (usually a serum protein such as albumin). The hapten molecule then acts as a determinant of antigenic specificity and is referred to as an **antigenic determinant**. Immunogens also have antigenic determinants which are simply particular chemical groupings within the macromolecule.

Specificity and cross-reactions
It is important at this point to distinguish clearly between structural specificity of an antigenic determinant and its distribution specificity. For example the ubiquitous nature of the glucose molecule — present in many different types of macromolecule — must be distinguished from its specific chemical structure. An immune response against a glucose determinant in antigen AG would be likely to react also with glucose in antigen BG provided the two determinants are equally accessible. The antibody directed against the glucose determinant is not, as is sometimes thought, a non-specific type of antibody but is simply reacting with an identical chemical determinant in another antigen molecule. A typical cross-reaction is with pneumococcal polysaccharide type S-VIII which has a tetrasaccharide repeating unit containing cellobiuronic acid alternating with an isomer of lactose. Antisera to such a structure will cross-react with oxidized cotton cellulose containing cellobiuronic acid residues.

Heterophile and Forssman antigens
In laboratory serological practice, **cross-reactions** are a common source of difficulty, and cross-reactivity is often found between antisera to certain bacterial antigens and antigens present in cells such as erythrocytes. Antigens shared in this way are known as **heterophile antigens** and antisera to these will cross-react with cells or fluids of many different species of animal and with various microorganisms. The chemical determinants responsible for this cross-reactivity are not known but are presumed to be similar or identical groupings possibly mucopolysaccharides and lipids present in large structural molecules. The best known of the heterophile antigens is the **Forssman** antigen which is present in the red cells of many species as well as in bacteria such as pneumococci and salmonellae. Another heterophile antigen is found in *E. coli* and human red cells of group B. Another important example is the cross reaction between *Treponema pallidum* and an extract of mammalian heart — **cardiolipin**. The common shared antigenic structures are phosphatidylglycerols differing only in their fatty acid side groups. Cardiolipin, being more readily available than *Treponema pallidum*, serves as a useful antigen in the serological test for syphilis (p. 239).

Carbohydrate, lipids, nucleic acids and protein antigens
It is common to classify antigens as proteins, polysaccharides or lipids; this is, however, an oversimplified view. Although many

molecules of entirely protein, polysaccharide or lipid nature are antigens, it is also not infrequent to find carbohydrate moieties as determinants on protein or lipid macromolecules or peptide units as determinants on polysaccharide macromolecules.

Carbohydrate determinants are commonly found in the cell wall of bacteria, and antibodies to these determinants are used for grouping the organisms. Streptococcal cell walls contain such antigens, and group A organisms have N-acetylglucosamine as the predominant determinant. In contrast group C streptococci have N-acetylgalactosamine as the main determinant. Pneumococci also contain polysaccharide in their capsules and the biological importance of these is discussed in Chapter 5.

Lipids and nucleic acids in purified form are not good at inducing an immune response and have to be complexed with a larger molecule or altered in some way before they do so. For example, nucleic acids conjugated to methylated bovine serum albumin can induce antibody formation. Nucleic acids as antigens are of some interest to immunologists as anti-nucleic acid antibodies are found in patients with the disease systemic lupus erythematosus (p. 215).

Proteins are highly complex molecules and have featured prominently in immunological studies because of their wide distribution in nature and their ready availability in highly purified form. Unfortunately, in the present state of knowledge of the antigenic determinants of protein molecules, so little information is available about the precise nature of the peptides acting as determinants in different protein macromolecules that immunologists still describe antigens in terms of the whole molecule, e.g. bovine serum albumin (BSA), rather than the individual determinants of specificity within the macromolecule.

Antigenic determinants

Degradation, chemical modification and synthesis of determinants
The number of determinants (sometimes referred to as its valency) in a molecule like BSA is probably in excess of 18 although only about six of these are exposed in the native intact molecule. The other (hidden) determinants can be identified only when the molecule is broken down by, for example, enzyme hydrolysis. Antibody produced in response to injection of the whole molecule appears to be able to react with the fragments produced by hydrolysis, and it therefore appears that the molecule is broken down into similar fragments after injection. This might be brought about by the digestive enzymes in phagocytic cells (p. 18).

Attempts to identify the chemical nature of antigenic determinants have used this type of degradation procedure with some degree of success and some insight has been gained into the size and other features of the determinants. Two other approaches have also been used — chemical modification of known determinants and synthesis of polyamino acid and polysaccharide antigens.

Degradation studies have been carried out on silk fibroin, a linear polypeptide chain of molecular weight between 50 000 and 60 000. The determinant site capable of reacting with antibody appears to consist of between eight to 12 amino acids 270–440 nm with the C terminal tyrosine making a considerable contribution to the site. The important role of **tyrosine** is further supported by the finding that the poor antigen gelatin can be made antigenic by the addition of tyrosine, in which the native molecule is very deficient. The posibility that tyrosine confers rigidity on the gelatin molecule has been suggested (see also p. 33).

The protein coat of tobacco mosiac virus consists of identical subunits (approx. 2000) each with a molecular weight of about 16 500 consisting of 158 amino acids. The antigenic determinant site is present in the chain between position 108 and 112 and, unlike fibroin, contains no aromatic amino acids. The hydrophobic nature of leucine appears to be an important characteristic of this particular determinant site.

The blood group substances are large molecules consisting of about 75% polysaccharide and 25% polypeptide. Degradation studies have shown that the substances owe their specificity to groups at the end of the carbohydrate chains, for example, A substances specificity is determined by α-N-acetylgalactosaminoyl-(1–3)-galactose.

Foreignness

A substance which acts as an antigen in one species of animal may not do so in another because it is represented in the tissues or fluids of the second species. This underlines the requirement that an antigen must be a **foreign** substance to elicit an immune response. For example, it follows that egg albumin, whilst an excellent antigen in the rabbit, fails to induce an antibody response in a fowl. The more foreign a substance is to a particular species the more likely it is to be a powerful antigen. A good antigen need not contain different building blocks, e.g. amino acids of a protein, but their arrangement should be such that at least part of the surface of the molecule present a configuration which is unfamiliar to the animal. Since macromolecules have a three-dimensional structure, it is easy to visualize how they could become unfolded by denaturation so as to present new and unique surface arrangements.

Foreignness can be a property which depends on chemical groupings which are entirely unfamiliar to the animals. Arsonic acid, for example, can be introduced by diazotization into a protein molecule. Such a group is known as a **hapten** and acts as the **determinant** of the **antigenic specificity** of the molecule, the protein to which the hapten is attached functioning simply as a **carrier molecule**.

Karl Landsteiner in the early part of this century carried out very extensive studies on the antigenic specificity of such hapten chemical determinants resulting in a new appreciation of how critical and precise was the fit between antibody and an antigenic determinant. Landsteiner's work with, for example, the arsonic acid determinant (AsO_3H_2) showed that changes, even as minor as the replacement in the benzine ring, of the AsO_3H_2 group by a COOH or a SO_3H group (Fig. 3.1) was sufficient to affect substantially the ability of azo proteins containing the determinant, to react with antibody against the unchanged hapten.

The influence of changes in shape brought about without the removal or substitution of groups is shown by studies with stereoisomers of macromolecules containing tartaric acid where the antibody to L-tartaric acid fails to combine with its isomer D-tartaric acid. It was concluded from studies of this type (a) that **acidic** and **basic** groups are very important in regulating the specificity of an antigenic determinant, (b) that **spatial** configuration of haptens is

Fig. 3.1 Rabbit antisera to azoproteins containing any of the above acid radicals as antigenic determinants react only with the inducing azoprotein and not with any of the others. Even azoproteins obtained by changing the — COOH of m-amino benzoic acid or the — SO_3H of metanilic acid to the ortho or para positions do not react with antisera to the original determinant. Methyl and halogen radicals substituted in the benzene ring instead of the acid radicals shown in the figure are less effective as determinants of specificity and considerable cross reactions are found in precipitin tests

important, (c) that **terminal** groups in an antigen are often important determinants of specificity and (d) that **interchange** of non-ionic groups of similar size had little effect on specificity of a determinant.

It became clear from studies of this type that a very slight variation in the chemical constitution or even shape of a molecule could substantially affect the ability of antibody to combine with it. Despite this knowledge immunologists even today are still far from understanding the chemical nature of the determinant groups in complex proteins and polysaccharides. Studies by Sela in Israel with synthetic polypeptides show that the **surface arrangements** of the amino acids in a branched polyamino acid structure are critical as determinants of antigenic specificity (Fig. 3.2).

If the three-dimensional structure of a protein is altered by heating or other form of denaturation, it is no longer able to combine as effectively with antibody to the original native molecule. Enzymes act as antigens and RNase molecules after oxidation become unfolded and the change in shape prevents the interaction of the molecule with antibody to native RNase.

■ Tyrosine   ◯ Glutamic acid   ▨ Poly amino acid backbone

Fig. 3.2 The amino acids, tyrosine, glutamic acid can convert a non-antigenic polyamino acid branched structure (polyalanine and polylysine) into an antigen provided they are attached to the outer end of the branches (left); if attached at the inner end of the branches (right) the complex is not antigenic

Immunogenicity

Molecular size

For a substance to be antigenic in its own right (i.e. an immunogen) without the need to be attached to a carrier molecule, requires that it has certain properties which have not yet been fully defined. Amongst these is the fact that **high molecular weight** materials are better antigens than those of low molecular weight but above a certain threshold it does not appear to be a determining factor. A substance below a molecular weight of about 5000 is not likely to be a good antigen. This phenomenon may be partly explained by the presence in a larger molecule of repeating antigenic determinant groups, and in a complex molecule of a large variety of potential determinants, one or more being capable of preferentially stimulating an immune response.

Large molecular size alone is not sufficient to confer antigenicity on a substance. Synthetic polymers of many types can be built up into large macromolecules and are non-antigenic. The polyamino acid backbone (polyalanine and polylysine) of the molecule shown in Figure 3.2 is non-antigenic and only becomes capable of inducing an immune response by the addition of further different amino acids. It has been suggested that the lack of antigenicity of synthetic polymers is due to their lack of internal molecular complexity. Thus the antigenicity of naturally occurring macromolecules may be due to their many different low molecular weight constituents giving complexity to the molecule. Tyrosine has been found to be a helpful constituent for a polypeptide to be a good immunogen although this amino acid is not essential. In general, aromatic amino acids consistently enhance the immunogenicity of a polypeptide.

Physical state, shape, charge

Some low molecular weight chemical substances appear to contradict the need noted above that an antigen be a large molecule. Among these are included picryl chloride, formaldehyde and drugs such as aspirin, penicillin and sulphonamides. These substances are highly antigenic, particularly if applied to the skin. The reason for this appears to be that such materials form **complexes** by means of covalent bonds with tissue protein, and the complex of these substances, acting as haptens with tissue protein carrier, forms complete antigen. This has important implications in the development of certain types of hypersensitivity states (p. 187).

The physical state of a protein antigen can affect its antigenicity. The same substance, e.g. the serum protein BSA, in aggregated and aggregate-free form can show wide divergence in ability to stimulate immunity, the aggregated form being strongly antigenic in the rabbit while the aggregate-free form induces a specific state of unresponsiveness (immunological tolerance, p. 87). This knowledge of the influence of **particle size** has been applied to production of antisera to snake venoms. The venom (neurotoxin) of low molecular weight and thus poor immunogenicity was linked to carboxymethylcellulose resin. The toxin-resin complex was non-toxic and highly immunogenic in rabbits.

Some molecules carry what is sometimes called 'built-in-adjuvanticity', which means that they have the capacity to stimulate the cells of the antibody system in a non-specific manner so that they are able to handle antigen more effectively. Bacterial endotoxin produces this effect as also do *Bordetella pertussis* organisms; these materials can enhance the antigenicity of a weak antigen if administered at the same time. The effect seems likely to be due to a powerful 'triggering' effect by bacterial endotoxin on a particular lymphocyte population (B cells, see p. 61) responsible for making antibody. In human immunization the efficacy of the 'triple vaccine', diphtheria, pertussis, tetanus, is partly due to the effect of *B. pertussis* (p. 141).

Polysaccharide antigen, for example dextran of molecular weight (MW) 600 000, is a good antigen, whereas a dextran of MW 100 000 is not. There is no obvious reason for this as the two materials are made up of identical building blocks and do not differ as far as the type of antigenic determinant is concerned.

The effect of electric charge of a molecule on its immunogenicity has been studied and found to be unrelated to its ability to induce an immune response. Polypeptides in which the net charge was zero elicited comparable amounts of antibody as charged polypeptides.

The shape of a polypeptide molecule does not affect its ability to elicit an antibody response and linear polypeptides which have no organized conformational structure can be potent immunogens.

Persistence of antigen
The ability of an animal to **degrade** a polysaccharide antigen can affect its immune reactivity to the antigen. Some pneumococcal polysaccharides appear to be resistant to digestion in the mouse and in sufficient dose are able to mop up antibody as it is made, resulting in the absence of detectable antibody in the serum. The same effect can be produced if the antigen is protected in some way from the tissue fluids and inflammatory cells. This can occur if the ma-

terial is incorporated in oil as an emulsion (see p. 61) or is walled off by fibrous tissue. The antigen dose, form, route of entry and host determinants are discussed in Chapter 4.

FURTHER READING

Barrett J T 1974 Textbook of immunology, 2nd edn. Kimpton, London
Borek F 1972 Molecular size and shape of antigens. In: Borek F (ed) Immunogenicity. North Holland, Amsterdam, p 45
Boyd W C 1963 Fundamentals of immunology. Inter-science, London
Dumonde D C 1965 Tissue-specific antigens. Advances in Immunology 5:30
Gill T J 1972 The chemistry of antigens and its influence on immunogenicity. In : Borek F (ed) Immunogenicity. North Holland, Amsterdam, p 5
Heidelberger M 1956 Lectures in immunochemistry. Academic Press, New York
Kabat E A 1968 Structural concepts in immunology and immunochemistry. Holt, Rinehart & Winston, New York
Landsteiner K 1945 The specificity of serological reactions. Harvard University Press, Cambridge, Mass.
Sela M 1965 Immunological studies with synthetic polypeptides. Advances in Immunology 5: 30
Sela M (ed) 1975 The antigens. Academic Press, New York

4

Acquired immunity

Objectives

On completion of this section the reader will able to:

1. Describe the two forms of adaptive immunity, humoral and cell-mediated

2. Outline the main determinants in the genetic control of immunity.

3. Differentiate between active and passive immunity

4. Starting with bone marrow stem cells, describe the development of the cells of the immune system

5. Describe the filtration and trapping function of the lymphoid organs and draw a diagram of their general structure

6. Briefly describe the evolution of the immune system

7. Differentiate primary from secondary immune response; consider time of response, types of antibodies produced, longevity of the response

8. List 3 determinants of acquired immunity

9. Give examples of the three main types of adjuvants

10. Draw a diagram of the IgG molecule; describe its possible evolution

11. List in the form of a table the five classes of immunoglobulin and their characteristic properties

12. Draw a diagram of the molecular structure of the IgG molecule and describe the functions of the individual domains

13. Define allotypes and idiotypes

14. Describe two selective transport mechanisms for immunoglobulins

15. List the cells concerned in the initiation of immunity and their characteristic surface markers and receptors

16. Outline the role of macrophages in the immune response

17. Define immune tolerance

18. Describe the role of T lymphocyte subclasses and how they are distinguished by differentiation antigens

19. Outline the subcellular processes involved in immunoglobulin synthesis by B lymphocytes

20. Define immunological memory

21. Describe the differences between selective and directive theories of immunity and outline the clonal selection theory

22. Describe the germline and somatic mutation hypothesis in the generation of antibody diversity

23. Describe lymphocyte transformation

24. List 10 lymphocyte activation products (lymphokines) and describe their main role in immunity

25. Briefly describe the role of the thymus in the immune response

26. Describe the main events in the cell-cooperative processes that lead to an immune response

27. Describe the routes of lymphocyte recirculation and the advantages of the recirculation process

28. Draw a diagram of the mouse MHC region and indicate the function of the different loci

Microorganisms which overcome or circumvent the innate non-specific immune mechanisms come up against the host's second line of defence. To give expression to this form of immunity it is necessary that antigens of the invading microorganisms come in contact with cells of the immune system (macrophages and lymphocytes), which leads to the initiation of an **adaptive immune response** specific for the inducing antigen. This response takes two forms, which usually develop in parallel and, although discussed separately, are closely related as both depend upon cells of the lymphoid system.

1. **Humoral immunity**. The characteristic of this form of immunity is the appearance in the blood of globulins known as antibodies or immunoglobulins. These combine **specifically** with the antigen which stimulates their production and can lead to some remarkable consequences. For example, the antigen molecules or particles may be clumped, their toxicity may be neutralised, their uptake and subsequent digestion by phagocytes facilitated and cellular antigens that are part of a cell surface such as a red blood cell or bacterium may be lysed.

2. **Cell-mediated immunity**. Lymphoid cells may be induced, by prior exposure to antigen, to react subsequently directly with the inducing antigen and bring about **cytotoxic** effects, as for example on foreign cells from a graft. The precise manner in which these sensitised cells perform this function is not understood and this is

an important area of current immunological research. This form of immunity is known as cell-mediated immunity.

General features

It is important to note that the immune response is a physiological reaction to the introduction into the body of **foreign** material, irrespective of whether it is harmful or not. Further, the response may be directed at antigens which are inside microorganisms and thus inaccessible to the serum proteins so that they perform no protective role. In contrast to innate immune mechanisms which vary greatly between species, the acquired response is little different between species and the main differences that can be detected occur between individuals.

The genetic control of the immune response

In 1938 Gorer and Schultze showed that there was a correlation between resistance to salmonella infections and the ability to produce antibody. Since this early work a large body of evidence has accumulated showing that the ability of an individual to respond to a particular antigen is under genetic control. There appear to be two forms of this control. (1) Control of the **general capacity** to produce an antibody response. This can be demonstrated by selective breeding of guinea-pigs or mice, which in a few generations can be divided into groups that give a uniformly good or a uniformly poor antibody response to several antigens. The poor response appears likely to be due to the slower mitotic division time of the responding cells. (2) Other genes are able to control the immune response to a **particular antigen** (e.g. a synthetic polypeptide in mice).

The genes controlling the ability to produce an immune response are called **immune response** or **Ir genes** and can be shown to be closely related in their position on a chromosome (number 17 in the mouse) to the genes controlling certain surface antigens of cells. These surface antigens are the major antigenic determinants in graft rejection (see Ch. 7, p. 161) and are called histocompatibility antigens.

The discovery of the immune response genes and their close linkage with the major histocompatibility antigen system in several animal species has given considerable impetus in recent years to a search for an association between susceptibility to a variety of neoplastic, autoimmune and infectious diseases and the activity of these genes. These associations are discussed in later chapters (p. 98 and 210).

Fig. 4.1

Active and passive immunity

An acquired immune state may be brought about in an individual in two main ways: (1) induced by overt clinical infection, inapparent clinical infection or deliberate artificial immunization. This is termed **actively acquired immunity** and contrasts with (2) **passively acquired immunity** which is transferred from an actively immunized individual to a non-immune individual by means of blood, serum components or experimentally by lymphoid cells.

Actively acquired immunity

Actively acquired immunity due to infectious agents falls into two general categories. Some infections, such as diphtheria, whooping cough, smallpox and mumps, usually induce a **lifetime immunity**. Others such as the common cold, influenza, pneumococcal pneumonia and bacillary dysentery, confer immunity for a shorter time, sometimes for only a **few weeks**. Failure of the second group of infections to induce lasting immunity is due to various factors, particularly to the fact that different members or strains of the same species of organism may be involved, and the acquisition of immunity to one strain does not prevent infection by another strain of the same organism.

The role of **nutritional factors** in the acquired immune response has been studied in experimental animals. Of the lymphoid organs the thymus appears to be affected the most, although the other lymphoid organs decrease in weight on severely restricted diets. The red pulp of the spleen and the lymphoid follicles are reduced in size. The absolute number of B lymphocytes are considerably reduced and is reflected in a failure of the lymph nodes to increase in cellularity on antigenic challenge with a consequent reduction particularly in the humoral response. Cell-mediated immunity may be less affected by poor nutrition, particularly in adults, because of the presence of long-lived recirculating lymphocytes (p. 96).

Passively acquired immunity

Administration of immune sera usually prepared in another species, e.g. the horse, is a therapeutic procedure in diphtheria and in gas gangrene. Antitetanus serum is used prophylactically when wounds may be contaminated with tetanus spores. Passive immunity may be conferred on the infant by the passage of maternal antibody across the **placenta** in some species such as the human and the rabbit, where a particular part of the immunoglobulin polypeptide chain has been found to be necessary for bringing about the transfer process (p. 74). In other species such as the rat and the dog antibodies are also transmitted in the **colostrum** to the intestine. Other animals, notably the lamb and the calf, receive this form of immunity only by means of the colostrum.

Pooled human immunoglobulin is also used as a source of antibody in a number of situations including measles infection and infectious hepatitis, when it is given during the incubation period to modify the attack. Human immunoglobulin is also given to patients with a congenital inability to make antibody globulin (p. 195).

ORIGIN OF THE CELLS OF THE IMMUNE SYSTEM — ONTOGENY

Haemopoiesis

The cells responsible for making the cellular components of the blood, a process called haemopoiesis, originate in the yolk sac of

Fig. 4.2 Simplified scheme of haemopoiesis and regulation

the embryo. They are found later in the fetal liver and later in the bone marrow. In the fully developed animal the bone marrow provides the haemopoietic stem cells from which arise the red cells, platelets, and leucocytes of the blood and tissues. These stem cells can be shown to be pluripotent, as by chromosome marker techniques, each of the cell types that develop from the stem cell can be shown to have the same chromosome marker and appear to be derived from identical stem cells.

The first stage of differentiation involving synthesis of DNA by the stem cell under the influence of various glycoproteins derived from mature leucocytes leads to the proliferation of a cell type called a progenitor cell. It differs from the stem cell in that it is responsive to hormone-like factors that lead to further differentiation. The progenitor cells, under the influence of chemotactic factors, seed the different lymphoid organs where the later stages of differentiation take place. These are called haemopoiesis-inducing microenvironments (HIMs). Certain epithelial cells in these microenvironments produce hormone-like factors which are thought to act on the progenitor cells to induce a particular pathway of differentiation. For example, differentiation towards erythrocytes in the microenvironment of the spleen under the influence of a factor called erythropoietin. Differentiation can occur towards certain lymphocyte types, e.g. thymic lymphocytes, in the thymus by a hormone called thymosin.

The process of differentiation is a continuous one because of the rapid turnover of blood cells. For example in man 1.6×10^9 neutrophils/kg of body weight are produced each day. There is great flexibility in the process so that even greater numbers of cells can be produced when required. The stimuli that lead to the production of these cells are very complex and not yet fully understood. They appear to involve what are called colony stimulating factors acting on the bone marrow stem cells. These factors are produced by blood leucocytes (including activated T lymphocytes p. 92), certain fetal tissues, and the placenta. The process can be modified to increased or decreased production by bacterial products such as endotoxin and various polysaccharide materials. Bone marrow damage by X-rays or cytotoxic drugs also leads to production of stem cell stimulating factors. The role of the colony stimulating factors in vivo has yet to be fully defined as have the environmental influences that enhance and suppress their production. The system has obvious physiological importance in the control of blood cell production including its ability to respond to inflammatory stimuli.

Lymphopoiesis

It is generally accepted that both B and T lymphocytes are generated from the pluripotent stem cell of the bone marrow. There are, however, many unanswered questions as to the detailed mechanisms involved. In particular, it is not clear how regulation is carried out or how the diversity of lymphocyte surface receptors is generated. The thymus gland has a critical role in T lymphocyte production as noted below, and this appears to involve thymic hormones. Regulation of B lymphocyte production in the bone marrow, and to some extent the spleen, is not understood. So far no regulatory factors have been found in the bone marrow microenvironment. The key step in the generation of B cell receptor diversity seems to take place by DNA rearrangement after B and T cell subclasses have been formed but preceding synthesis of messenger RNA, and, therefore, before immunoglobulin is produced. It is thought that the stem cells resemble germ line cells and are not restricted with respect to the specificity of receptors that their progeny can produce.

The role of the thymus in immune reactivity

Development and structure. The thymus in mammals arises from the endoderm of the third and fourth branchial clefts and is the tissue in which lymphocytes can first be recognised. The thymus gland increases in size until puberty and then slowly atrophies although it is still readily recognizable in the adult. The cells of the thymus are of three main types: **thymocytes** morphologically similar to blood lymphocytes, **phagocytic reticulum cells** and **reticular epithelial cells**. The macroscopic structure of the organ is like that of other lymphoid organs in general organization, with a central medulla containing a high proportion of reticular cells and a peripheral cortex containing the thymocytes with some surrounding reticular cells. Unlike the spleen and lymph nodes there are no germinal centres and no plasma cells. Thus under normal physiological conditions the thymus cells do not make antibody. Plasma cells will appear only if antigen is injected directly into the organ. Hassall's corpuscles are a feature peculiar to the medulla of the thymus and consist of groups of reticular epithelial cells sometimes flattened and concentrically arranged around a central core of nuclear debris.

Cell turnover and humoral factors. The thymus can be shown, by tritiated thymidine incorporation studies, to be actively engaged in lymphopoiesis, there being a higher proportion of primitive actively dividing lymphoid cells than in any other lymphoid tissue such as the spleen or lymph nodes, and with a correspondingly high mitotic rate. Evidence suggests that the stimulus for thymocytes to divide arises in some way from the reticular epithelial cells. The primitive cells in the thymus are slowly replaced during life by cells derived from the bone marrow that migrate via the bloodstream into the thymus. A small proportion of these cells leave the thymus and find their way to the peripheral lymphoid tissues; these are the **long-lived lymphocytes** with a life of months in rodents and possibly years in man.

Maturation of T cells during the period they spend in the thymus has been shown to take place. The changes associated with this can be detected by means of **membrane antigens** on the T lymphocytes. The main murine antigen markers are known as Thy (theta), TL and Ly antigens. The TL antigen is present on the lymphocytes that enter the thymus but is lost on maturation in the gland. The amount of Thy antigen is also much reduced during this period and the Ly antigens develop and are expressed on mature T lymphocytes. Various functional characteristics have been found to be associated with different Ly antigens and T lymphocytes carrying such antigens can thus be divided into **subpopulations**. The functional activities that can be defined on the basis of Ly markers are 'helper cell activity' (see cell cooperation, p. 45), cytolysis of allogeneic lymphocytes or tumour cells, i.e. 'cytotoxic T cells' and 'suppressor cell' activity involved in controlling B lymphocytes. Suppressor T cells in the mouse are characterised by surface markers (differentiation antigens) and are susceptible to thymectomy, X-irradiation, and cyclophosphamide. Suppressor cells express differentiation antigens, the Ly-2 and Ly-3 antigens as well as antigen coded by the I–J subregion (see p. 98 and Fig. 4.25). Helper T cells express Ly-1 antigen. About 60% of Ly-1 cells express an additional antigen, the Qa antigen, coded by a locus close to the H-2D end of the MHC complex in the mouse (Fig. 4.25). The Ly-1 Qa^+ cells appear to control the generation of suppressor cells, probably by means of effects on a third subpopulation of lymphocytes expressing Ly-1, 2, and 3 antigens that themselves exert feedback inhibition of the Ly-2 suppressor cells.

The regulatory circuits are very complex as are the experiments designed to elucidate their details. In simple terms, the Ly-1 cells can be thought of as the central lymphocyte population, rather like C3 in the complement system. These cells act to screen the surface of other cells, particularly macrophages, for foreign materials associated with MHC molecules. When such foreign material is 'seen' by the Ly-1 cells, they induce a variety of effector cells to make a specific immune response and at the same time act on resting T cells causing them to emit various stimulatory and inhibitory stimuli. For a more detailed description of these complex regulatory mechanisms, the reader is referred to the references under Further Reading. Table 4.1 shows the various cell functions that appear to be associated with each of the differentiation antigens.

Table 4.1 Functions associated with differentiation antigens

Differentiation antigen	T cell type	Cell function
Ly-1	T_h	Helper T cell Stimulation of B cell probably through macrophage.
	T_d	Transfer of Delayed Hypersensitivity
Ly-2,3	T_s	Suppressor T cell acting on T_h cell
	T_c	Cytotoxic T cell (type 1 reactions)
Ly-1,2,3	? Immature T cell	Acted upon by T_h cell carrying Qa antigen and then controls T_s activity

If the thymus is removed during the neonatal period, it is possible to find lymphocyte-deficient areas in the white pulp of the spleen around the central arterioles and in the paracortical area of the lymph nodes. These areas have been termed the '**thymus-dependent**' areas of the lymphoid tissues. Associated with this localised deficiency of lymphocytes, neonatally thymectomised animals also have considerably impaired cell-mediated immune effector mechanisms affecting graft rejection and other forms of cell-mediated immunity such as delayed hypersensitivity reactions; humoral immune reactivity is much less markedly affected.

Studies in mice of cell turnover in the adult thymus show that the thymic population of lymphocytes is replaced every three or four days but that the great majority of cells never leave the organ and die there. The reasons for this **intense lymphopoiesis** is unknown. In the adult it seems that the thymus is necessary for repopulation of lymphoid tissues depleted by X-irradiation or other methods. However, studies with chromosome markers have shown that the new cells are not derived directly from the thymus but are lymphoid cells from elsewhere in the body, probably from the bone marrow. The role of the thymus in this situation appears to be the production not of thymus-derived cells but of a humoral factor, **thymosin,** which restores immunological reactivity to remaining lymphoid cells. This was strongly suggested by experiments in which thymus implants in millipore diffusion chambers were placed in the peritoneal cavity of thymectomised mice. Immunological capacity was restored to the recipients, which recovered the ability to reject skin grafts, although the chambers were impermeable to cells and were on later recovery shown to contain only reticular epithelial and reticulum cells and no lymphocytes.

The essential functions of the thymus can be summarised as bringing about the **differentiation** and **proliferation** of primitive bone marrow-derived lymphoid cells and producing a **humoral factor** with the ability to induce immunological competence in lymphocytes. Immunologists are unfortunately as yet some way from understanding fully the exact mechanisms of interaction between the gland and the peripheral lymphoid tissues.

It is worth noting at this point that the hormonal factor produced by the thymus is not the only hormonal influence acting on the lymphoid tissues. **Growth hormone** increases thymus weight and thyroid hormone increases the weight of the lymphoid tissues and the size of the immune response. Adrenalectomy also increases the weight of the lymphoid tissues, and **glucocorticoids, oestrogens** and **androgens** decrease its weight. After neonatal thymectomy acidophilic growth hormone producing cells of the anterior pituitary appear to lose their granules suggesting an increased demand for output of hormone by the cells in the absence of the thymus. Interference with the production of **anterior pituitary** hormones in mice by means of specific antisera results in lymphocyte depletion in both thymus and spleen. All these observations indicate the close relationship between endocrinological function, immunological maturation and expression of immune capacity.

CELL COOPERATION

Central and peripheral lymphoid tissues
Knowledge of immune-reactivity which is either thymus-dependent or bursa-dependent has led to the concept of separate **central** and **peripheral** lymphoid tissues. The central organs — the thymus and the bursa of Fabricius (or its equivalent in mammals, initially fetal liver and later bone marrow) — are responsible for development and control of the peripheral lymphoid tissues — the spleen and lymph nodes.

A tentative scheme showing the possible inter-relationships of central and peripheral lymphoid tissues is given in Figure 4.4. Experimental work, based on repopulation of irradiated animals by lymphoid cells from different origins, indicates that for the expression of at least some forms of immune response, there is co-

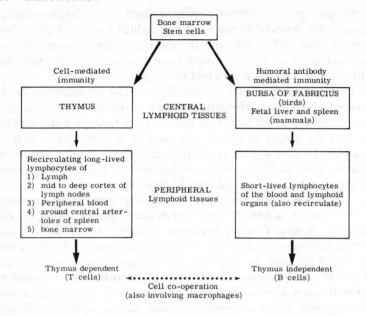

Fig. 4.3 Scheme illustrating possible relationship between central and peripheral lymphoid tissues

operation between cells in the peripheral lymphoid tissues derived directly from the bone marrow and lymphocytes derived from the thymus. The former cells are referred to as **B cells** (bone marrow derived) and the latter as **T cells** (thymus-dependent). The B cells are responsible for **immunoglobulin synthesis** and may sometimes be directly stimulated by contact with antigen — usually powerful antigens such as salmonella flagellin or haemocyanin. Other weaker antigens such as serum albumin require the co-operation of T cells acting as **helper cells** leading in some way to an immune response by the B cells. T cells and macrophages may, for example, concentrate antigen and present it to B cells, or perhaps T cells may release soluble factors (p. 92) to stimulate B cells (see p. 77 and section on cell co-operation and genetic control, p. 98). T and B cells are morphologically indistinguishable until they transform after antigenic stimulation. The cytoplasm of transformed T lymphocytes can be seen under the electron microscope to contain numerous polyribosomes; in contrast the transformed B cell is packed with rough endoplasmic reticulum followed by the appearance of intracytoplasmic vesicles of antibody (p. 83, Fig. 4.20). Both T and B cell populations show a similar change in their behaviour after primary and secondary antigenic stimulation the cell populations. Both increase in size and develop immunological memory. Initially the B cells produce IgM antibody and then switch to IgG production; coincident with this change the surface receptors on these B cells change from IgM to IgG type (see p. 83).

T lymphocyte receptors

There is much discussion among immunologists about the nature of the receptor for antigen on T lymphocytes. Immunoglobulins that resemble the monomeric subunits of IgM have been isolated from T lymphocytes. Their detection depends upon incorporating a radioactive label into the membrane immunoglobulin. Released labelled immunoglobulin can then be detected in the culture medium of the T lymphocyte preparations. The immunoglobulin detected in this way appears to have a particular ability to attach to cells thought to be macrophages. It is suggested that this T cell immunoglobulin assists in the initiation of the immune response by trapping antigen on the macrophage surface, where it is presented to B cells that are then triggered to produce antibody. Not all immunologists are convinced that the 'T cell immunoglobulin' (sometimes called IgT) is actually produced by the T cell but that it may be taken up passively after being produced by B lymphocytes. However, certain T cell lines kept in culture are claimed to actively synthesise a T cell immunoglobulin, but it remains to be established if this is an in vitro artefact not reflected in normal T lymphocyte populations in vivo. Other T cell products of non-immunoglobulin nature have been described which appear to assist B cells to respond to antigen and this is discussed on p. 92.

Recent work on the **genetic control** of the immune response (see p. 98) has provided evidence that the antigen binding site on T cells is closely linked to (or even part of) a product of the gene complex controlling the histocompatibility antigens of the cell membrane.

It has already been noted (p. 43) that T cells express receptors which recognise products of the major histocompatibility complex on other lymphoid cells, such recognition being essential for cell cooperation in the immune response. Work with rats and mice indicates that the T cell receptor expresses the same idiotype (i.e. the antigenic determinants found in the antigen binding site of the Fab fragment, p. 69) as serum antibodies of the same specificity. The conclusion from these and similar experiments is that T cell receptor structure is coded for by immunoglobulin genes for the variable portion of the heavy chains (p. 68).

B lymphocyte development

The details of the regulation of B lymphocyte differentiation from pluripotent stem cells is not as well understood as those of the T lymphocytes.

Gut-associated lymphoid tissue and antibody production

The thymus appears to control the cells of the cell-mediated immune system (p. 90) probably by providing facilities for the maturation of immature bone marrow cells. The cells of the immune system concerned with producing circulating antibodies reside mainly in the cortico-medullary junction and medullary cords of lymph nodes and the red pulp of the spleen.

The first evidence that B lymphocytes might be influenced by a non-thymic lymphoid organ came from phylogenetic studies in neonatal chickens which failed to develop normal immunological capacity after removal of the gut-associated lymphoid organ known as the **bursa of Fabricius**. Thymectomised chickens, as would be expected from the discussion above, fail to develop cell-mediated immune processes whilst capable of a humoral immune response. In striking contrast, bursectomised chicken fail to make immunoglobulins and have no plasma-cells or germinal centres in the lymphoid organs. Their cell-mediated mechanisms are, on the other hand, intact. Evidence is now emerging which suggests that there is a traffic of bursal lymphocytes to germinal centres in the spleen and lymph nodes comparable to that described in the thymus for bone marrow lymphocytes.

In mammalian species immunologists have been searching for years for an organ equivalent to the bursa in birds. After a few false leads indicating the possible involvement of gut-associated lymphoid tissue of the appendix and Peyer's patches, it was found that the bone marrow is the specific microenvironment where B cells differentiate from stem cells. Some 80% of the marrow small lymphocytes are of the B cell lineage. So far a hormone-like regulatory molecule responsible for B lymphocyte differentiation has not been identified. The immature rapidly dividing B cell precursors have μ heavy chains, characteristic of IgM (p. 69), but no light chains in their cytoplasm. There is a particular gene family in the chromosome of the B cell line for each of the two types of light chain, λ and κ, and a third for the various types of heavy chain. The three loci are unlinked and in the mouse are found in chromosome 6 and 12. The B lymphocyte family or clone that develops from a single stem cell is able to switch the expression of one type of heavy chain to another without changing the part of the molecule containing the amino acid sequences that bind antigen, the variable region (p. 67). The earliest form of B cell (pre-B cell) is detectable in the fetal liver and bone marrow. It can synthesise IgM but this is found only in the cytoplasm; it appears later in the membrane, 16 to 17 days in mice and 9 days in man. The μ chain of the molecule as it appears in the membrane of the B cell is slightly different chemically from the secreted form of IgM. This seems to depend on there being two forms of μ mRNA derived from a single gene. The membrane form of the μ chain is 21 amino acids longer than the secreted form and contains uncharged hydrophobic amino acids that are thought to anchor the μ chain in the membrane.

A similar mechanism seems likely to operate also with each of the other immunoglobulin heavy chains but this has yet to be established. The diversity of amino acid sequences found in the part of the molecule that combines with antigen (variable region) is thought to be controlled by somatic mutation which is discussed more fully on page 89.

The immature B cells leave the bone marrow and migrate to the secondary lymphoid tissues. At the same time surface IgM increases in density. During this period the B cells can become tolerant. Various other receptors become detectable: Fc, Ia and C3 receptors, and IgD begins to appear. These changes are independent of exposure of the B cells to antigen. The IgD is lost on antigenic stimulation. The mechanism underlying the switch to production of other classes of immunoglobulins is not understood. It is not clear whether this depends on antigenic stimulation or can occur only under the influence of microenvironment factors (see also pp. 74, 83).

THE TISSUES INVOLVED IN SYNTHESIS OF ANTIBODY

The lymphoid tissues which are predominantly engaged in the immune response are the **lymph nodes, spleen** and **bone marrow**. Whilst the lung and to a lesser extent the liver can both take part in the immune response, their contribution is much less than that of the other tissues. The large overall contribution of the bone marrow is a reflection of the mass of this tissue throughout the skeleton. However, weight for weight the spleen and lymph nodes by far exceed the capacity for antibody production of the bone marrow. For this reason much effort has been expended in attempting to unravel the way in which the specialised lymphoid organs, the spleen and lymph nodes take up foreign antigens and initiate the immune process.

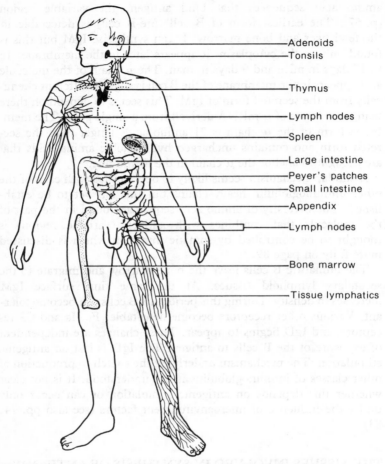

Adenoids
Tonsils
Thymus
Lymph nodes
Spleen
Large intestine
Peyer's patches
Small intestine
Appendix
Lymph nodes
Bone marrow
Tissue lymphatics

Fig. 4.4 Tissues and organs of the immune system. Human lymphoid system: lymphatic vessels collect interstitial fluid from extremities and carry lymphocytes and foreign materials to draining lymph nodes to initiate an immune response. Lymphatic vessels also leave lymph nodes and carry recirculating lymphocytes to neck veins to enter bloodstream. Lymphocytes leave blood via capillaries and via specialised blood vessels in the lymph nodes and spleen and recirculate. This allows recruitment of lymphocytes at sites of inflammation, replenishment of lymphoid organs if existing lymphocytes are destroyed by, for example, X-rays or infectious agents, and enables lymphocytes to have access to antigens anywhere in the tissues. Diagram also shows the bone marrow of a long bone from where the stem cells derive that develop into cells that populate the lymphoid organs (lymph nodes and spleen). Some of these stem cells, before entering these organs, pass via thymus gland and become thymus-derived or T lymphocytes. The respiratory and gastrointestinal tract have collections of lymphoid tissue — tonsils and adenoids of the oropharynx and Peyers patches and appendix of the intestine. The lymphoid tissues are filtering systems to remove foreign antigens from the bloodstream and lymph and where immune responses usually occur. (Reproduced from Blackwell C C, Weir D M 1981 Principles of infection and immunity in patient care. Churchill Livingstone, Edinburgh, p 61)

The role of the thymus gland and co-operation between different cell populations in the early events preceding antibody synthesis will be described later in this chapter.

The spleen, lymph nodes, bone marrow and other lymphatic tissues that engage in antibody production are **vascular filtration systems**. They depend on a three dimensional network of reticular cells and reticular fibres. In these filters, **antigen** is **trapped** and **cells** become lodged from the circulating blood and lymph and can **interact, differentiate** and **proliferate** in the organ.

Figure 4.4 gives an overall view of the distribution and location of the tissues and organs of the immune system.

Gross structure
The **lymph nodes** of the human are structures of the shape and approximate size of a bean. In smaller animals they are of the same general structure but correspondingly smaller. The lymph flows from the limbs and organs through the lymph nodes on its way to the main lymphatic vessels of the neck and their union with the veins. The afferent lymphatics enter the capsule of the node (Fig. 4.5) and the lymph leaves via the efferent lymphatics of the hilum. Trabeculae extend radially into the node from the capsule, passing from the marginal lymph sinus through the cortex to the medulla. The tissue of the gland consists of a meshwork of reticular cells in which large numbers of **lymphocytes** are embedded. These cells are grouped in nodules or **follicles** in the cortex and form in-

ROUTE OF ANTIGEN

Germinal centre with rim of lymphocytes. Cells at centre are actively dividing cells, cells at periphery are antibody forming.

Afferent lymphatic

Primary follicle

Cortex

Paracortical area (Mid-deep cortex, Thymus dependent)

Medulla

Marginal sinus

Efferent lymphatic

Fig. 4.5 Lymph node

terconnected cords in the medullary area sometimes called medullary cords. Around each nodule in the cortex is a condensation of reticular cells. A reticular network provides a scaffolding for the lymphocytes, makes up the sinuses and supports the blood vessels and nerves. A nodule that enlarges after antigenic stimulation is termed a **germinal centre** and includes macrophages with cytoplasmic extensions or dendritic processes. **Macrophages** are present throughout the gland, many being found in the medullary area. **Plasma cells** and their precursors are also found, particularly at the cortico-medullary junction. Arteries enter the node at the hilum and their capillaries end up in post-capillary venules with a tall lining endothelium. Between and through these endothelial cells blood lymphocytes pass into the node.

The **spleen** (Fig. 4.6), like the lymph nodes, is enclosed by a capsule and divided by trabeculae into communicating compartments. The organ plays an important role in destruction of **red cells** and their production; as well as producing **platelets, granulocytes** and **lymphocytes**. Its major immunological role is to act as a filter for the bloodstream. The tissue consists of (a) the **white pulp** — around the branches of the splenic artery which are surrounded by periarterial lymphatic sheaths and lymphatic nodules or Malpighian bodies, and (b) the red pulp — splenic sinuses and splenic cords, the latter making up bands of tissue, reticulum cells, erythrocytes, lymphocytes and granulocytes — lying between the sinuses which are themselves lined by 'sinus-lining cells' held together by a network of reticular fibres. The blood leaves the white pulp via capillaries and enters the red pulp passing into the

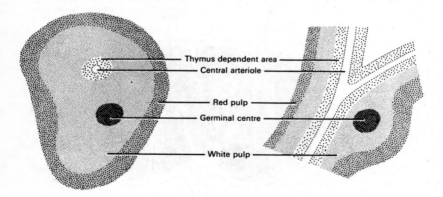

Thymus dependent area
Central arteriole
Red pulp
Germinal centre
White pulp

Fig. 4.6 Structure of Malpighian corpuscle. Tranverse section of part of spleen showing area of white pulp related to central arteriole and considered to be thymus-dependent sinuses and is collected up into venules and veins leaving by the splenic vein. The precise details of the blood circulation in the spleen are not yet fully elucidated, but particulate material and cells can clearly pass through the walls of splenic vessels or be discharged directly into the splenic tissue (p. 97). It can thus be seen that the lymph nodes and spleen can be regarded as a complex organization of three types of cell involved in the initiation of the immune reaction — lymphocytes, plasma cells and phagocytic cells of the mono-nuclear phagocyte system.

This account of the structure and histological detail of the spleen and lymph nodes must not obscure the fact that many of the cells in these organs are part of a mobile population circulating between the blood and lymphoid tissues (p. 96).

Development

The lymphoid tissues responsible for humoral antibody production are associated developmentally with the gut and consist of lympho-cytes and plasma cells of the lymph node and spleen. The lymphoid tissues responsible for cell-mediated immune reactivity are associated with the thymus (see pp. 42–45 for further discussion on this subject). In both the spleen and lymph nodes there are areas of lymphoid tissues under the influence of the thymus — the so-called **thymus-dependent areas** (Fig. 4.6) — lying adjacent to the central arterioles in the spleen and the post-capillary venules in the medulla of the lymph node. After experimental neonatal thymectomy these areas do not develop properly and cell-mediated immune reactions are absent. There is a rare human condition. (Di George's syndrome, p. 199) where this occurs in the absence of thymus function. Histo-logical examination of the spleen and lymph nodes shows that the areas described are deficient in cells.

In the humoral immune response, immunoglobulins are secreted into the blood by lymphoid cells — predominantly **plasma cells** situated in the spleen and lymph nodes. In contrast the cell-mediated response when it occurs peripherally (e.g. in the skin) is effected by migration of the stimulated cells themselves from the lymphoid tissue via the efferent lymphatics to the bloodstream. Some of the cells leave through the capillary endothelium to pass into the tissue fluids where they are ready to interact with for-eign antigenic material. These cells are then collected by the afferent lymphatics and recirculate (p. 96).

Organised lymphoid tissues are **absent in invertebrates** and the most primitive of the vertebrates, the hagfish. This system develops late in phylogeny and the first traces appear in the lamprey. Both these primitive vertebrates are, however, able to show a limited degree of adaptive immunity. Their serum contains a primitive form of immunoglobulin that appears to be related to IgM (see below), which has since become considerably diversified. The amphibians are the most primitive animals to show IgG, and all species higher in the evolutionary scale than birds have IgM, IgG and IgA.

The precursors of the early immunoglobulins are likely to have arisen in the prevertebrate era although as yet there is no direct evidence for this. It has been suggested that they may have arisen from receptors on the surface of phagocytes which enable the cells to distinguish foreign material from self. It seems possible that such receptors could have the molecular properties of the combining site of an antibody molecule (see below).

The **complement system** appeared some time later in evolution and is developed in the jawed vertebrate, the paddle fish. With increasing structural complexity of animal species the immune reaction has become more diversified and effective. However, once components of the immune system appear in evolution they are maintained with a remarkable constancy both at the molecular and functional level.

In the human, lymphoid tissue appears first in the thymus at about eight weeks' gestation. Peyer's patches are distinguishable by the fifth month and immunoglobulin secreting cells appear in the spleen and lymph nodes at about 20 weeks. From this period onwards both IgM and IgG globulins (p. 65) are synthesised by the fetus with IgM predominating. At birth the infant has a blood concentration of IgG comparable to, or sometimes higher than, that of maternal serum, having received IgG but not IgM via the placenta from the mother (p. 74). The rate of synthesis of IgM in the infant increases rapidly within the first few days of life but does not reach adult levels until about a year. This compares with the much slower rise in IgG and IgA globulins which do not reach adult levels until between the sixth and seventh years of life. Cell-mediated immune reactions can be stimulated at birth but these reactions (e.g. homograft rejection) may not be as powerful as in the adult, although the evidence for this is rather scanty.

Invertebrate immunity

For many years it had been generally assumed that the adaptive immune response was a characteristic of the vertebrates and that invertebrates lacked the ability to mount an immune response. The recent recognition of a limited ability in the most primitive of the vertebrates, the hagfish, to exhibit cell-mediated immunity, suggests that the origins of the immune response may well have been rather earlier. Immunologists are now exploring the possibility that invertebrates can produce at least some form of adaptive immune response.

Specific recognition by certain primitive marine organisms (coelenterates) of the cells of unrelated species is a well-documented phenomenon and can be seen in colonial hydroids, gorgonians and reef-building corals. **Rejection of grafts** shows convincing specificity, but no immunological memory leading to accelerated rejection on second exposure has been demonstrated.

Invertebrates have a well developed **non-specific** cellular defence mechanism to cope with foreign materials that enter its tissues. The process is mediated by blood cells called **haemocytes** which phagocytose the foreign particle and localise it in a fibrous nodule. This process is quite distinct from the cell-mediated immune response of vertebrates as it does not result in the formation of a descendant family or clone of cells with a specificity limited to the inducing agent (see Fig. 4.7). Evidence has, however, been obtained in work with annelids and echinoderms showing that they are capable of rejecting grafts from unrelated members of the same species. On repeated grafting **accelerated rejection** takes place indicating the development of what could be a secondary immune response. It seems

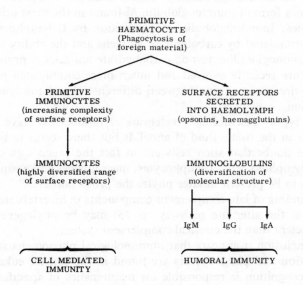

Fig. 4.7 Schematic view of proposed stages in evolutionary development of adaptive immune response

clear that the mechanism underlying this rejection process is quite distinct from the non-specific haemocyte response to any foreign substance and may well turn out on further study to be a form of specific adaptive immune response.

The tissue fluids of invertebrates have been known for many years to contain a variety of **agglutinins** for vertebrate eythrocytes. These haemagglutinins can be shown to act as **opsonins** (p. 73) facilitating phagocytosis. Many attempts have been made unsuccessfully to increase the quantity of these haemagglutinins in the tissue fluids by immunization of invertebrate species (e.g. in crayfish). Of some interest is the finding that the natural haemagglutinin of the horseshoe crab is a protein of molecular weight of approximately 400 000 consisting of 18 subunits of 22 500 each. The subunits have a molecular weight comparable to that of a vertebrate light chain and some similarity in their amino acid composition. These findings have led to the suggestion that the haeagglutinin may represent the product of a primitive form of light chain gene.

Some recent work indicates that certain invertebrate agglutinins are **specific** for cell wall **carbohydrate** determinants, e.g. N-acetyl D galactosamine and N-acetyl neuraminic acid. These findings have potentially important implications for understanding of the evolution of the immunoglobulins of higher animals. The precursor of these was a form of immunoglobulin M found in the most primitive vertebrates. Immunoglobulin M production by B lymphocytes is readily stimulated by carbohydrate antigens and the ability to produce immunoglobulins to non-carbohydrate antigens is probably a much more recently evolved and much more complicated process that requires co-operation between different cells of the lymphoid population.

Cell types resembling vertebrate lymphocytes have been observed in the tissue fluid of annelids but there seems to be considerable doubt that such cells are in fact the precursors of vertebrate lymphoid cells. Lymphocytes, macrophages and eosinophils do seem to be present in later phyla, the protochordates.

The finding of late complement components in invertebrates suggests that the alternate pathway (p. 23) may be phylogenetically more ancient than the classical complement system.

In conclusion it appears that immunological phenomena such as **recognition** and **phagocytosis** are found in the earliest eukaryotic cells. Recognition is responsible for maintenance of **specific partnerships** in metazoa, for exclusion of potentially harmful **microorganisms** and perhaps also for removal of altered or dead tissue constituents. **Cellular immune mechanisms,** such as rejection of un-related tissue cells (initially without immunological memory), is a feature of all eukaryotic animals and precedes the development of humoral immunity. The emergence of organised lymphoid tissues occurred in the early vertebrate era and immune mechanisms be-came increasingly efficient with the development of cooperative re-lationships between the different cellular elements.

THE IMMUNE RESPONSE

Immunoglobulin production — the humoral antibody response
The antibody response resulting from exposure to antigenic sub-stances has certain well-defined characteristics. After first meeting the antigen there is an interval of about two weeks before antibody can be found in the blood, and during this initial period there is in-tense activity in the antibody-forming tissues. This can be shown by studies with isotope-labelled precursors of cell components, for example tritiated thymidine, to show DNA synthesis or carbon-14 labelled amino acids in protein synthesis. Following antigenic stimu-lation there is a rapid increase in cell proliferation and synthesis of protein in the cells of the lymphoid organs indicated by the in-corporation of the labelled materials. If the lymphoid cell popu-lation of a rat is depleted by placing a cannula in the thoracic duct and draining off the lymph, then no such cell proliferation takes place and there is no antibody response. In contrast in a normal animal immunised, for instance with sheep red blood cells, lympho-cytes taken from the spleen or lymph nodes can be shown to have synthesised anti-sheep cell antibodies. If sheep red cells are mixed with the spleen or lymph gland cells the red cells aggregate around individual lymphocytes giving a rosette appearance when examined microscopically (Fig. 4.8). The red cells become attached to the surface of lymphocytes by means of antibody located at the cell membrane.

The antibody which eventually can be detected in the blood — the so-called **primary immune response** — does not reach a high level and does not persist unless a second dose of antigen is given (Fig. 4.9). When this happens, any remaining antibody will be rapidly mopped up by combination with the antigen and this will be reflected by a fall in detectable antibody in the blood; then after only a day or two a remarkable rise in the level of antibody begins and reaches a peak shortly thereafter which can be from 10 to 50 times higher than the primary response. This **secondary response** is maintained at a high level, falling only slowly over a period of

IMMUNO-CYTO-ADHERENCE
Rosette technique

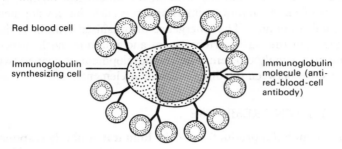

Red blood cell

Immunoglobulin
synthesizing cell

Immunoglobulin
molecule (anti-
red-blood-cell
antibody)

LOCALISED HAEMOLYSIS IN GEL
Jerne Plaque technique

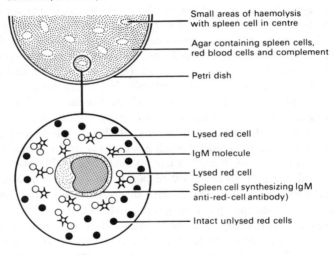

Small areas of haemolysis
with spleen cell in centre

Agar containing spleen cells,
red blood cells and complement

Petri dish

Lysed red cell

IgM molecule

Lysed red cell

Spleen cell synthesizing IgM
anti-red-cell antibody)

Intact unlysed red cells

Fig. 4.8 Two methods for demonstrating antibody formation by single cells. In the immuno-cyto-adherence test spleen cells from an animal immunised with, for example, sheep red blood cells, are mixed with the red cell antigen and after a period of incubation 'rosettes' are formed as shown. The red cells often completely surround the antibody-producing spleen cells. In the Jerne plaque technique, the spleen cells from the sheep-cell immunised animal are mixed with the red cell antigen in soft agar and when complement (guinea-pig serum) is layered on the surface, lysis of the red cells occurs. This happens because the antibody produced by the spleen cell has diffused into the surrounding agar and coated the red cells. This enables the complement system to be activated with the resulting lysis of the red cell (see p. 23 for the description of complement lysis)

months. The response can be boosted to even higher levels by further injections of antigen until a stage is reached when no further increase occurs. It is important to note that once an animal has responded to an antigen, even though exposed to it on only one

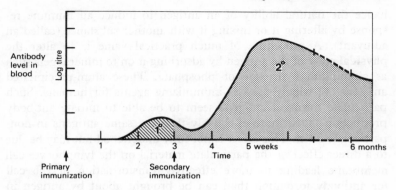

Fig. 4.9 The antibody response

occasion, the animal retains a **memory** of the antigen so that even after an interval of months or years it is able to react by means of a secondary response with a rapid mobilization of antibody-forming cells. Hence vaccination against an infective agent such as smallpox or poliomyelitis virus provides many years of useful protection against infection, even though soon after vaccination the level of antibodies falls to a low level, since the memory has been retained.

To obtain a maximum response, the **interval** between the primary and secondary injections should not be too short and an interval of less than 10 days is likely to reduce the level of the secondary response; subsequent injections should be spaced out to weeks, then to months (p. 141). This allows time for the increase in numbers of antibody-forming cells which can be stimulated by subsequent injections. The lymphocytes engaged in the initiation of humoral antibody production are derived from the bone marrow and are referred to as **B cells**. This cell differentiates into the main antibody synthesising cell — the **plasma cell**. The characteristics of this cell population are discussed later in this chapter.

Some of the host determinants of acquired immunity have already been mentioned. The nature of the antigen, the form in which it is presented, the route of injection and the dose given also have marked effects on the response.

Determinants of acquired immunity

Form, dose and route of entry of antigen
The determinants of antigenic specificity have been discussed above (p. 30), as have the effect of molecular weight and the need for foreignness of the antigenic material. It is, however, possible to en-

hance the natural ability of an antigen to induce an immune response by altering it or mixing it with another substance (called an adjuvant). A procedure of much practical value is to alter the **physical state** of the antigen by adsorbing it on to mineral gels such as aluminium hydroxide or phosphate. These alum-precipitated antigens are widely used as immunizing agents for humans. Such particulate forms of antigens seem to be able to initiate antibody production much more effectively than the same antigens in non-particulate form. This effect is not fully understood but may be due to a direct effect of the particulate material on the lymphocyte cell membrane leading to more effective transformation of the cell for antibody formation than can be brought about by antigen in solution.

An additional factor which may be important for some types of antigen is that particulate material is more readily phagocytosed by macrophages. These cells have been shown in certain situations to make a contribution by serving as a store of antigen for later release and stimulation of lymphocytes. It has been suggested that macrophages may also improve the antigenicity of weak antigens by altering them in some way before passing them on to lymphocytes. It is conceivable also that by removing antigen from the circulation they protect the lymphocytes from the effects of excess antigen which would be likely to paralyse the lymphocytes rather than initiate antibody production (p. 80). For a protein antigen a dose of a few hundred microgrammes is required to stimulate the production of detectable circulating antibody. The increase in antibody response is small in proportion to the increase in dose of antigen given and is approximately proportional to the square root of the increase in antigen administered until an upper limit is reached. An increase above this level can, as indicated above, result in specific paralysis of the antibody-forming tissues. This form of inhibition, sometimes referred to as **immunological tolerance,** is specific only for the antigen which brought it about. The lymphoid tissues remain normally responsive to other antigens.

Other methods have been developed to enhance the antibody response, although at present they are used mainly in experimental work. The most important of these consists of the preparation of a **water-in-oil emulsion** (Fig. 4.10): an aqueous solution of antigen is emulsified in a light mineral oil so that tiny drops of antigen solution are dispersed throughout the oil. The emulsion forms a depot of antigen in the subcutaneous tissues from which small quantities of antigen are continually released, sometimes for a year or more. An influenza vaccine in this form has been used successfully in

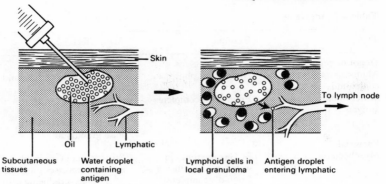

Fig. 4.10 Water in oil adjuvant (depot forming adjuvant)

man. New possibilities have been opened up by the development in Edinburgh of a multiple form of emulsion, in which the aqueous solution is first dispersed in oil and the oil is finally dispersed in a water phase. These emulsions are stable and much less viscous and less difficult to inject that the water-in-oil type. An even better response is achieved if killed tubercle bacilli are included in the emulsion; a wax constituent of the bacterial wall is responsible for this effect. The bacterial product appears to stimulate the cells involved in the immune response. Such emulsions are of course only suitable for experimental work and are often termed **Freund's** adjuvants after their originator.

The advantages of these **adjuvant** methods of immunization are that both the primary and secondary immune response are achieved by only one injection of antigen and that the peak level of antibody is maintained over a long period by the small quantities of antigen released from the depot.

Table 4.2 gives a list of examples of the three main types of adjuvant that are used: **depot** or **repository, bacterial** and **chemical**. The main effects of these adjuvants on the immune system (where known) are shown in the table. In the last few years adjuvants have been widely employed in tumour immunotherapy, both in experimental animals and man, and this is discussed further on page 177).

If an antigen is given intravenously most of the antibody is produced by the spleen, and some in the lung and bone marrow; on the other hand, if given subcutaneously or intradermally, the antigen travels via lymphatics to the local lymph nodes where antibody production is initiated. When antigen is given with adjuvants, there is a local accumulation of inflammatory cells, and antibody pro-

Table 4.2 Adjuvants

Type	Example	Main effects
Depot or repository		
Aluminium and calcium compounds	Aluminium phosphate	Slow release of antigen and local granuloma
Water in oil emulsions of antigen	Freund's incomplete	Slow release of antigen, emulsion droplets carry antigen to lymph nodes, local granuloma
Bacterial		
Mycobacteria	BCG (sometimes in water-in-oil emulsion — Freund's complete)	Stimulation of macrophage activity, increases numbers of antibody-producing cells
Anaerobic coryneforms	*Corynebacterium parvum*	Stimulation of macrophage activity, augmentation of certain classes of immunoglobulin e.g. IgM. Immunostimulation for antibody responses and immunosuppression of cell-mediated immune responsiveness.
Bordetella	*B. pertussis*	Activation of macrophages, lymphocytosis (shift of lymphocytes from T and B cell areas of lymphoid tissues)
Bacterial polysaccharides	various Gram negative organisms	Activation of lymphocytes
Chemical		
Lysolecithin analogues	C_{18} ether hydroxy lysolecithin	Activation of macrophages
Lysozome labilizers	Vitamin A, beryllium salts silica	Activation of macrophages
Polyanions	Double stranded, natural and synthetic polyribonucleic acids	Increase numbers of memory cells, activation of T lymphocytes and macrophages (interferon production)
Fungal polysaccharides	Lentinan (a glucose polymer)	Not known (possible stimulation of T lymphocytes)
Imidazole derivative	Levamisole	Not known

duction occurs in the resulting granulomatous tissue as well as in the draining lymph nodes.

THE IMMUNOGLOBULINS

Enormous advances have been made in the last decade in knowledge of the chemical structure of immunoglobulins and the relationship of the **structure** to the **biological activities** of the molecule. These have enabled immunologists to agree internationally on a nomenclature which distinguishes a number of different classes of immunoglobulin on structural rather than functional characteristics. It was the practice to refer to an antibody as an agglutinin, a neutralizing or a precipitating antibody, when it was not realized that each of these activities could be exhibited by a chemically heterogeneous population of molecules and could be shared by the same molecule. Other classifications were dependent on the behaviour of the molecules in electrophoresis, which did little more than split the population up into still heterogeneous groups of proteins differing in their overall charge and molecular size.

Methods have been developed in America for the fragmentation of the immunoglobulin molecule by chemical cleavage in Edelman's laboratory, and by pepsin digestion by Nisonoff. Porter in Britain was the first to achieve cleavage with retention of biological activity of the fragments using papain digestion. These studies gave impetus to the work which now has enabled immunologists to distinguish five main classes of immunoglobulin each based on a similar polypeptide chain structure consisting of two pairs of 'heavy' and 'light' chains joined by disulphide bonds sometimes occurring as multiples of this basic unit.

It is considered that the molecule is based on a **12-unit structure**, each unit or domain consisting of a polypeptide chain with 110 amino acids of MW 12 000. Each light chain of MW 25 000 consists of two of the basic units and each heavy chain four basic units. Heterogeneity of immunoglobulin structure occurs within this general framework with some of the basic units being affected more than others. Figure 4.11 shows a tentative view of how the mol-

Fig. 4.11 Possible evolution of the immunoglobulin molecule

ecule may have evolved from the basic unit, perhaps arising as a receptor on a phagocytic cell. The ancestral molecules, consisting of a single domain that immunoglobulin may have evolved from, are β2 microglobulin and Thy-1. These molecules form part of the array of substances found on the surface of various tissue cells. β2 microglobulin is a component of certain histocompatibility glycoprotein antigens and these are known to be involved in recognition of similarities and differences between cells. The evolutionary advantage provided by antibody-like molecules has ensured their maintenance and diversification over hundreds of millions of years. A picture of the immunoglobulin molecule has been built up and is

Fig. 4.12 Diagrammatic view of structural arrangements of polypeptide chains of immunoglobulin molecule. The chains are held together by three disulphide bonds. Pepsin splits the molecule, leaving an Fc fragment (crystallizable) and Fd parts of the heavy chains with attached light chains — the whole making Fab (or antigen binding) fragments. The N terminal ends of the light and heavy chains have variable sequences of amino acids as shown by the broken line. There are also a number of intra-chain disulphide bonds which influence the shape of individual chains. The carbohydrate (Cbh) groups may be concerned with the catabolism of the molecule

represented in Figure 4.12. The general arrangement has been confirmed by electron microscopy.

On the basis of marked **antigenic differences** in the **heavy chains** it has been possible to define **five classes** of human immunoglobulin, using the technique of immunoelectrophoresis. These are referred to as IgG, IgM, IgA, IgE and IgD (Table 4.3) (Fig. 4.13). IgM seems to have been the first immunoglobulin molecule to evolve. IgG and IgA probably evolved from the IgM by loss of single basic unit (domain) from the heavy chains (see below).

Immunoglobulin G or IgG

This is the major immunoglobulin component of serum making up 75% of the total and having a molecular weight of 160 000 in the human. The molecule has two antigen-binding sites as shown in Figure 4.12 on what are termed the **Fab** portions of the molecule and involving part of both the heavy and light chains. The amino acid sequences have been worked out in whole or in part for a small number of light and heavy chains in various species, using myeloma proteins which are present as a homogeneous population in the serum of individuals with plasma cell tumours in sufficient quantity to enable studies of this type to be made.

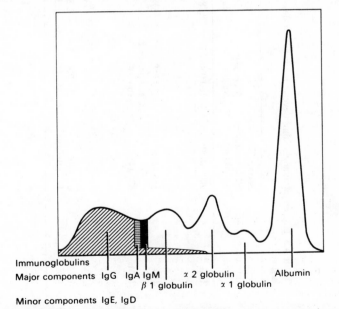

Fig. 4.13 Electrophoretogram obtained by UV scanning of paper electrophoresis strip and showing diagrammatically the main components of human serum and the immunoglobulin classes

Table 4.3 Human immunoglobulins (levels vary widely, males tend to have slightly lower levels of IgG and IgM but higher IgA)

Immunoglobulin class	Serum concentration mg/100 ml	Molecular weight	Half life days	Light chains	Heavy chains	Characteristic properties
IgG	900–1800	160 000	18–23	K and L	γ	Precipitins Antitoxins Complement fixation
IgA	156–294	170 000 and polymers	5–6.5	K and L	α	Late antibody Surface protection
IgM	67–145	960 000	5	K and L	μ	Agglutinins Opsonins Lysins, complement fixation
IgD	0.3–40	184 000	2.8	K and L	δ	Early antibody Not known
IgE	10–130 (μg)	188 105	2.3	K and L	ε	Reaginic antibody

The light chains can be shown to consist of two parts joined together. One has a **constant** sequence of amino acids at the C terminal end of the chain, common to the light chains of the species under study. The other part is at the N terminal end in which **variation** occurs in the sequence of the 107 amino acids. The variable portion differs between one myeloma and another, being similar only within a particular myeloma. Up to 50% of the positions in the N terminal portion have been found to be variable. This leads to an enormous number of different permutations of sequence and thus in antibody specificity. An animal may have a repertoire of a thousand different V_L and V_H regions that between them can account for up to a million potential antibody specificities. The other domains, one in light chains and 3 or 4 in heavy chains, make up the constant or C region. Similar variation has been found in rather more limited studies of the N terminal end of the **heavy chain**. The variable portions of the light and heavy chains are contained in the Fab portion of the molecule and it is in this **variable portion** of the chain that the **antigen-binding** site is present.

More recently, as larger numbers of immunoglobulins have been sequenced, it has become apparent that the amino acid variability tends to be concentrated in three so-called **hypervariable** regions. The remaining amino acid sequences of the variable regions, when one immunoglobulin is compared with another, fall into V region subclasses (four for K chain V regions and five for L chain).

The discovery of V region subclasses demonstrates that V region sequences have been more **strictly conserved** during evolution than that of the constant regions. No species-specific amino acid residues have so far been found in the variable portion and this suggests that during embryogenesis a single gene controls the development of the entire range of variability in the light chains. This gene probably arose early in evolution and the survival value associated with diversification of the antigen-binding site has ensured its maintenance since then.

The **light chains** are of two distinct types known as K or L (κ or λ) chains. In any one individual, both K and L chains are produced but they are not found together in the same immunoglobulin molecule. K and L chains are present in a ratio of about 2:1 in any one individual. Two intra-chain disulphide bonds (Fig. 4.12) occur in almost exactly the same position in both K and L chains and both chains have cysteine as the terminal amino acid at the carboxyl end. This serves for the attachment to the heavy chains. These facts suggest a **common genetic origin** of K and L chains which, although they have **diverged** during evolution, have retained many common structural characteristics.

The **heavy chains** are specific for each class; in the human IgG molecule the heavy chain or γ chain exists in four different forms, IgG1, IgG2, IgG3 and IgG4, which can be distinguished by specific antisera able to detect differences in the Fc fragment of the heavy chains. Sixty-five per cent of the IgG molecules in human serum are of the IgG1 subclass, 23% of the IgG2 and 8% and 4% IgG3 and 4. Differences have been found in the numbers and position of the disulphide bonds in the different IgG subclasses and these are shown diagrammatically in Fig. 4.14. Disulphide bonds are essential to the normal 3-dimensional structure of immunoglobulin molecules and differences in their location may be reflected in different biological activities.

The separate immunoglobulin chains consist of repeating homologous units called **domains**; two for light chains, four to five for heavy chains (μ and ε heavy chains have five). A so-called 'hinge' region occurs on heavy chains of all classes except IgM. It is inserted between the Fd and Fc portions and contains the inter-heavy-chain disulphide bridges. The domain at the amino terminal end of each H and L chain is the variable or V region referred to above and is the part which recognizes and binds foreign antigens.

The domains show many **homologies** in their amino acid sequences and were probably derived from an ancestral gene coding for the length of one domain. This gene was presumably doubled then redoubled and, within each resulting gene, crossing-over and mutation has since led to the differences that can now be detected in their products. The further back in evolution that divergence between the genes took place, the fewer the similarities. The generation of subclasses is relatively recent in evolution and there is therefore a high degree of homology.

Fig. 4.14 IgG subclasses showing variable arrangements of the disulphide bonds

Individuals can be subdivided on the basis of certain characteristics of their immunoglobulin molecules. These are comparable to the blood groups but instead of involving antigenic differences in the surface antigens of red cells, they depend on antigenic differences in the light and heavy chains of the immunoglobulin molecule. These genetically determined sub-groups are known as **allotypes**. Three main groups, Gm, Km and Am, have been found and each can be subdivided. The antigenic determinants of the Gm groups are carried in the γ chains of the IgG molecule only. In contrast the Km factors are present in the K light chains of each of the immunoglobulin classes. Am allotypes have been found in the IgA2 subclass.

The variable portions of the heavy and light chains of the Fab fragment have also been shown to carry antigenic determinants. These depend on the amino acid sequences in the variable portion that determine the specificity of the antibody. Thus Fab fragments of different specificity have different antigenic determinants. These are called **idiotypic** determinants and are characteristic of the particular clone of cells producing a specific antibody and have proved of considerable value to immunologists as a way of following the activity of a particular clone of cells by identifying the idiotypic marker. Isotypes also exist and are due to antigenic determinants on all molecules of a certain class or subclass of heavy chains or of certain light chains.

IgM, IgA and IgD
Like IgG globulin each of these classes of immunoglobulin in man has been found to contain K and L light chains. The heavy chains, on the other hand, are unique for each of these types of immunoglobulin, IgM containing μ chains. μ chains have five subunits or domains (one variable and four constant) compared with four subunits in γ and α heavy chains. IgE (see p. 184), like IgM, also has an extra domain in its ε heavy chains. IgA have α chains and IgD δ chains and it is these differences which enable them to be distinguished one from another. There are two subclasses of IgA (IgA1 and IgA2). IgA2 is unusual in that the light chains are linked to each other by disulphide bonds instead of to the heavy chains (they are linked covalently to the heavy chains in this subclass). IgA1 accounts for 90% of the total serum IgA in contrast to secretions, where IgA2 makes up as much as 60% of the total. IgM globulin, with a molecular weight of about 900 000, can be split by reduction of disulphide bonds into five subunits. These subunits have a

molecular weight of 180 000 and are believed like IgG to have two heavy and two light chains.

Until recently most studies on the number of antigen-binding sites of IgM antibody showed that the molecule had only five binding sites despite the fact that theoretically 10 were present. Both human and rabbit IgM however have now been shown to have the 10 sites and it is believed that the two binding sites on each are unable to combine with antigen with similar efficiency thus making it difficult to demonstrate all 10 sites. Polymeric forms of IgA and the IgM molecule have recently been shown to have a small polypeptide called the J chain.

This polypeptide has a molecular weight of about 15 000 and differs in structure from all known immunoglobulin polypeptide chains. It is rich in cysteine residues and appears to exist in a molar ratio of one J chain per polymer regardless of how many immunoglobulin subunits make up the polymer. The J chain makes up about

Fig. 4.15 IgM structure showing five subunits and multiple combining sites

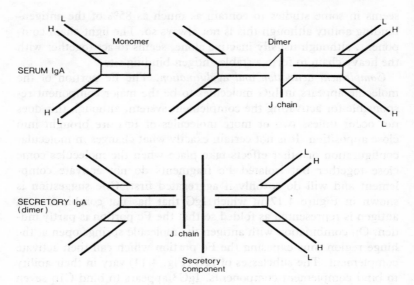

Fig. 4.16 IgA showing monomer, dimer and secretory form, with J chain and secretory component

1% of the IgM molecule by weight and in the IgA molecule about 3%.

The role of the J chain is not entirely clear but the fact that it is added at the final polymerisation stage just before the molecule is secreted at the cell membrane of the synthesizing cell suggests that it may be required in the secretion process. It is noteworthy that IgM subunits are not found free in the serum, although polymers of IgM without J chain are found in certain pathological conditions. The role of the J chain in the IgA molecule may be to activate the transport molecules that carry IgA through the mucous membranes and may perhaps be responsible for the ability of the IgA molecule to bind secretory piece (see p. 74). The molecular structure of some of these immunoglobulins is shown in Figures 4.15 and 4.16.

Structure and function of immunoglobulins

Knowledge gained from the structural studies discussed above has helped towards an understanding of the biological activities of the immunoglobulin molecule and it is now possible to pinpoint areas of the molecule responsible for different activities. The areas of the light and heavy chains (Fab portion) containing the variable sequences are the site of that part of the molecule with the capacity to combine with antigen. The heavy chain component (Fd portion) seems in some studies to contain as much as 85% of the antigen-binding ability although this is not always so. The light chain component, although usually inactive alone, seems to act together with the heavy chain to form a stable antigen-binding site.

Complement activation and agglutination. The Fc portion of the molecule appears in IgG molecules to be the major component responsible for activating the complement system, although this does not occur unless two or more molecules of IgG are brought into close apposition. It is not certain exactly what changes in molecular configuration or other effects take place when the molecules come close together but isolated Fc fragments do not activate complement and will do so only if aggregated first. One suggestion is shown in Figure 4.17 in which IgG that has not combined with antigen is represented as folded so that the Fc portion is partly hidden. On combination with antigen the molecule springs open at the hinge region thus exposing the Fc portion which can then activate complement. The subclasses of IgG (Fig. 4.14) vary in their ability to bind complement components. IgG3 appears to bind C1q seven times more effectively than IgG1 and IgG4 does not bind complement at all.

It has been calculated that a single IgM molecule attached to a red cell by its multiple combining sites can bring about lysis whereas 1000 IgG molecules are required for the same effect. Humphrey and Dourmashkin, who came to these conclusions, assumed that as two IgG molecules must come together for complement activation, a large number of IgG molecules would be required for this to occur as the antigenic determinants are spread evenly over the surface of the red cell. Agglutination is brought about by the linking of particulate antigens such as red cells or bacteria by the two Fab fragments of the immunoglobulin molecule.

As might be expected from knowledge of the structure of the IgM molecule, its five combining sites make it a very efficient

Fig. 4.17 Possible molecular forms of IgG before and after combination with antigen (see text)

agglutinating antibody molecule and rabbit IgM antibacterial antibody is known to be 22 times as active as IgG antibody (mol/mol) in bringing about bacterial agglutination. Because of its large molecular size IgM is largely confined to the bloodstream and probably plays an important role in protection. Deficiency of IgM is often associated with susceptibility to septicaemia. IgG antibodies on the other hand are more effective than IgM antibodies at neutralising diphtheria toxin, lysozyme or viruses such as poliovirus. Whilst some of this activity was present in isolated Fab fragments, the evidence from virus neutralisation indicates that the Fc fragment may assist the Fab fragments in neutralisation of virus infectivity. The molecular basis for such effects has yet to be elucidated.

Tissue fixation and opsonisation. The ability of immunoglobulin to attach to tissue cells appears to be a well-marked feature of the IgE class of immunoglobulin responsible in humans for various forms of hypersensitivity reaction (p. 184) and may be dependent on the activity of the Fc portion of the molecule. This is suggested by studies of the ability of immunoglobulin fragments to adhere to guinea-pig skin and produce a particular form of hypersensitivity reaction that is known as passive cutaneous anaphylaxis. Immunoglobulin antibody specific for particulate antigens such as bacteria plays a valuable role by coating the surface and making the antigen more susceptible to phagocytosis. These are known as opsonising antibodies and IgM antibodies perform this role particularly efficiently. In the rabbit it has been shown that IgM anti-salmonella antibodies are some 500 to 1000 times more effective than IgG antibodies as opsonising agents.

How opsonisation is brought about is not clear; it is possible that antibody may alter the surface properties, such as the surface charge of a particulate antigen, and thus perhaps reduce electrostatic repulsion between phagocyte and antigen. It also can be shown that the Fc fragments of the antibody have an affinity for the surface of the macrophage and thus link the particulate antigen (attached by means of the antibody combining sites) to the macrophage (attached by the Fc fragment). Antibody with the ability to attach to macrophages by means of the Fc fragment has been described in the guinea-pig and is known as cytophilic antibody. Antigen-antibody complexes appear to be localised in the lymphoid follicles of lymph glands due to the activity of the Fc portion of the immunoglobulin molecule.

The presence of immunoglobulin molecules as receptors for antigen on the surface of lymphocytes has been confirmed by a variety of techniques. B lymphocytes can clearly be shown to have light chains and heavy (μ) chains on their surface, but the situation as far as T cells are concerned is less clear (see p. 47).

Recent work indicates that IgD is present on the majority of B lymphocytes in the cord blood of human infants and in a lesser proportion of adult B lymphocytes. The molecule does not cross the placenta and is absent from cord serum. The significance of these observations is not yet clear. A similar immunoglobulin has been found in the mouse and occurs together with other classes of immunoglobulin on a substantial proportion of B cells in the spleen, lymph nodes and Peyer's patches. Immature B cells (uncommitted) appear to have μ (IgM) heavy chains and later to develop δ (IgD) chains in addition. At a later stage in differentiation δ and γ (IgG) chains are formed without μ chains.

Selective transport. The newborn animal, emerging from an environment where it has been sheltered from antigenic stimuli, is protected by maternal immunoglobulins transmitted from the mother. These antibodies often reach a level higher than in the mother and persist longer in the circulation of the young animal than they would do in the adult. This transferred **passive immunity** tides the infant over the period until its own immunological system begins to mature.

In humans, IgG globulins can pass through the placenta and reach the fetal circulation; this is not a simple filtration process, but is due to selective transfer of the molecules involving a part of the Fc fragment of IgG heavy chains. This property is a feature only of the γ heavy chains of IgG and has not been found in the μ and α chains of IgM and IgA. This mechanism seems to be limited to **primates** whilst in **ruminants** maternal immunoglobulins from the colostrum reach the fetus through the intestinal epithelium.

Another selective transport mechanism is found with IgA globulins which are selectively secreted into saliva and respiratory and intestinal **mucous secretions** as well as into the **colostrum**. The site of synthesis of IgA is in submucosal plasma cells of the **lamina propria** of the gastrointestinal tract and in the salivary glands and mammary glands. In the lamina propria of human gastrointestinal tract the IgA-producing cells outnumber the IgG cells by about 20:1 in contrast to lymph nodes and spleen where the ratio is 1:3 (IgA:IgG). The IgA found in mucous secretions is manufactured as a dimer with a J chain component and has an attached **secretory** or transport piece not found except in small amounts in serum IgA. It seems likely that it is added to the molecule during its passage into the mucous secretions from the lamina propria, underlying the mucous membrane of the gut and respiratory tract. The secretory component has a molecular weight of 70 000, the J chain 15 000 and the secretory IgA is an 11S molecule of molecular weight 400 000. The IgM present in secretions has also been found to have secretory component bound to it, whilst any IgG or IgE found in secretions does not. About 4% of the plasma cells of the respiratory and gastrointestinal mucosa are making IgE and, like IgA-producing cells, contribute to serum IgE levels.

In contrast to other immunoglobulins, salivary and colostral IgA, probably because of the attached secretory piece, appear to be relatively resistant to digestion by proteolytic enzymes. This would clearly be an advantage in allowing this immunoglobulin to remain active and able to perform a protective role in the intestinal tract. The dimer form of IgA gains the ability to fix complement and after attaching to Gram-negative organisms there is evidence that the activation of the complement system by the IgA may allow the enzyme lysozyme (p. 15) to digest the mucopolysaccharides of the microorganism's cell wall. Much effort is being expended by laboratory workers in studying the role of IgA as a protective mechanism at the mucous surface and the possible future use of vaccines designed to stimulate this form of antibody response may be of considerable value.

An interesting suggestion has been made, supported by some experimental evidence, that IgA in the mucous secretions may inhibit the binding of potentially pathogenic microorganisms to the mucous membranes and thus prevent infection. IgA may play a role by combining with food constituents that could act as allergens and prevent their passage through the gut wall. This idea is supported by the finding that infants with reduced serum IgA levels soon after birth seem more likely to develop allergic states at about 1 year of age. See page 120 for further discussion of IgA activity.

THE CELLS CONCERNED IN ANTIBODY PRODUCTION

Antigen localisation and contact with macrophages and lymphocytes
A simplified picture of the cellular mechanisms leading to antibody formation is that antibodies of different specificities are made by different families or **clones** of cells, each family being genetically programmed to make antibody of only **one specificity**. There is evidence to show that the cells carry at least part of the molecule of their particular antibody exposed on the cell membrane as a receptor for antigen. Thus when an antigen is injected into the body and comes in contact with lymphoid cells it combines with those ex-

posed antibody receptors which are best able to fit the determinant groups of the antigen molecule.

The way this is brought about can be seen when isotope-labelled antigen is injected into an animal. It is first rapidly localised in the sinus-lining macrophages in the marginal zone around the Malpighian bodies in the spleen or the medullary macrophages of the lymph nodes (Fig. 4.5), depending on the route of injection (p. 59). After this localisation, plasma cell precursors (probably small lymphocytes) at the cortico-medullary junction of the lymph nodes are triggered to proliferate and differentiate into antibody-producing cells; exactly how this triggering mechanism works is not yet understood. One possibility is that after partial degradation in the macrophage, antigenic fragments are passed on to the lymphocytes. It is also possible that some antigens can react directly with the lymphocytes themselves (see below). This stimulation and proliferation lead to the development of lymphoid follicles, which are localised collections of active lymphoid cells taking part in the primary immune response.

Subsequent contact with antigen now results in a rather different pattern of localisation influenced by the presence of secreted antibody to the antigen; antigen, whilst still taken up by medullary macrophages, is also localised on the surface of **dendritic macrophages** (macrophages with cytoplasmic extensions) which interdigitate with each other and with the lymphoid cells of the lymphoid follicles or Malpighian bodies. This localisation seems to depend on antibody at the surface of the macrophage. Lymphocytes themselves may also come directly in contact with antigen. They can be shown to have at least portions of the immunoglobulin molecule on their surface because they can readily be stimulated to respond by transformation, to contact with antibodies directed at various parts of the immunoglobulin molecule. The specificity of these surface immunoglobulins is thought to be determined by the **genetic constitution** of the particular lymphocyte. Nossal in Australia was able to isolate single antibody-producing cells in a 'microdroplet' and show that such cells taken from an animal immunised with salmonella produced only one type of antibody. It has been inferred from this that the cell receptor and the secreted antibody are of the same specificity and it has been found that receptors can only be seen clearly on the antibody secreting cell population (i.e. the B cells).

Immunoglobulin heavy chains are present as a component of the immunoglobulin receptor on B cells; they are μ chains as found in IgM and the molecule appears to be an IgM subunit (similar in MW to IgG and called IgMs). B lymphocytes prior to antigenic stimulation are believed to synthesise around 250 to 5000 subunits of IgM per hour per cell. The molecules are shed from the surface membrane into the extracellular fluid.

The B cell membrane possesses **receptors** for the Fc fragment of the immunoglobulin molecule and a receptor for the activated complement component C3. It is not yet clear what role these receptors play in B cell activity. The possibility has been suggested that binding of activated C3 leads to B cell activation and that the Fc receptor acts as a receptor site for IgM molecules, in particular subunits of IgM (IgMs), which appear to be the predominant immunoglobulin present on B cells. Another suggestion, based on the ability of antisera directed against histocompatibility antigens to block uptake of labelled complexes of antibody and antigen, is that the Fc receptor is related to the product of the immune response (Ir) genes and that the receptor may be involved in the genetic control of immune responsiveness by B cells. The detailed mechanisms underlying these proposals are as yet far from being resolved and await a much clearer understanding of the histocompatibility gene complex and its products as represented in the cell membrane.

Microscopic examination of lymphocytes exposed to antigen has shown that antigen tends to bind preferentially to certain areas of the lymphocyte membrane rather than uniformly over the cell surface. The surface immunoglobulin receptors seem to be able to **coalesce** at points around the cell membrane, suggesting that they have a degree of mobility. This finding is consistent with current views on the structure of cell membranes indicating that they are made up of a lipid bilayer containing protein molecules that can move around, coalesce and separate when for example the pH of the surrounding medium is changed.

Properties of antigen, cell co-operation and activation of lymphocytes
Binding of antigen to the immunoglobulin receptors on a B lymphocyte, whilst a necessary prelude to activation of the cell for immunoglobulin synthesis, is not in itself sufficient to ensure B cell stimulation. For successful activation the antigen molecule must have additional properties, rather like the mitogenic properties of phytohaemagglutin (see p. 91), which provide a **'signal'** to activate the cell.

Certain antigens, e.g. bacterial lipopolysaccharides, have this property and can stimulate B cells unaided. Other antigens, e.g. serum proteins, although able to bind to the B cell, are unable to deliver the activating 'signal'. These latter antigens require the assistance of T lymphocytes to **co-operate** with the B lymphocyte and provide the necessary stimulus for activation.

The observations that led to these conclusions allowed the identification of two categories of antigen: (1) those that bind and activate B lymphocytes without the assistance of T lymphocytes, referred to as **T-independent antigens**, and (2) those that can bind to B lymphocytes but require the co-operation of T lymphocytes for B cell activation, referred to as **T-dependent antigens** (Fig. 4.18).

A number of hypotheses have been put forward to explain how B cell stimulation is achieved; they fall into two categories — the so-called 'one signal' and 'two signal' models. One signal models propose that B cells can be triggered by antigens with repeating antigenic determinants that cross-link adjacent immunoglobulin receptors on B cells. The T cell in this model is believed to function as a regulator of B cell function — **suppressing** or **stimulating** according to the needs of the situation. Two signal models propose that two specific signals must be delivered to the B cell in order for triggering to occur. Signal 1 is delivered by binding of antigen to the immunoglobulin receptor on the B cell, and Signal 2 by a T cell product or perhaps by a macrophage product (see below). One proposal by Feldman is that the T cell produces a specific immunoglobulin in response to part of the antigen molecule (carrier

Fig. 4.18 Scheme showing how T-independent and T-dependent antigens trigger B lymphocytes to synthesise antibody. Macrophage products may be responsible for activating T lymphocytes (see p. 79) and macrophages themselves may present antigen to B cells (not shown in diagram)

portion) and that this immunoglobulin (IgT) is cytophilic (i.e. binds) for macrophages. The macrophages then bind antigen and present it to B cells leading to triggering and antibody formation.

Direct presentation of antigen to B cells by T lymphocytes has been proposed, perhaps in the form of antigen bridging between the two cells. The T cell binds antigen by receptors that recognise determinants on the protein molecule that carries within it smaller (haptenic) determinant groups with which B cells can interact (but not respond to without T cell cooperation). This effect is called the **carrier effect** and was originally shown using haptenic groups such as dinitrophenol (DNP) attached to a protein carrier like bovine gamma globulin (BGG) or ovalbumin (OA). T cells appear to recognise the carrier and B cells the hapten. An animal immunised to DNP-BGG would not respond to a subsequent challenge with DNP-OA, indicating the need for T cells to recognise the carrier before B cells could respond to the hapten.

It seems probable that B cell activation and antibody synthesis can be the end result of a number of different stimuli, and that **macrophages, B cells** and **T cells** may all contribute in varying degrees, depending on the nature of the antigen, the dose of antigen and its mode of presentation.

The role of macrophages in antibody production
Macrophages play an important role in the **initiation of the immune response** by T and B lymphocytes. It has been known for some years that macrophages are required in order to obtain an im-

Table 4.4 Cells concerned with initiation of immune response

Cell	Essential functions
Macrophages	Remove and catabolise excess antigen
	Localise and retain antigen at 'critical sites' and present antigen to lymphocytes
	Regulate activities of lymphocytes by soluble factors
	Bind antigen-antibody complexes by Fc and C3 receptors
T lymphocytes	Act as 'helper' cells for certain antigens (T-dependent)
	Regulate activities of macrophages and B lymphocytes and recruit other T lymphocytes by soluble factors
	'Production of 'IgT' cytophilic for macrophages for presentation of antigen to B lymphocytes
B lymphocytes	Immunoglobulin production
	Binding of antigen by Ig receptors and responding to T-independent antigens. Fc and C3 receptors binding antigen-antibody complexes and possible role in activating the B lymphocytes and regulating their activity

mune response to sheep red blood cells by mouse spleen cells in vitro, and these findings have since been confirmed with a number of antigens and in different species. The source of the macrophages was found to be important, and whilst those from the spleen or peritoneal cavity were effective, macrophages from the lung (alveolar macrophages) and liver (Kuppfer cells) were not able to co-operate with lymphocytes in the initiation of an immune response. The latter cells do, however, possess many features — functional and morphological — of macrophages, including the ability to adhere to glass, to phagocytic particles and to be cytotoxic for antibody coated cells.

Immune responses induced in vitro in spleen cell suspensions suggest that the macrophage appears to be necessary for an immune response to occur to T-dependent antigens (see above) and its presence has been shown to be necessary for the triggering of B lymphocytes by at least some T-independent antigens. Exactly how the macrophage helps in the processes leading to antibody production is not clear but the 'sticky' surface properties of the cell and its ability to take up antigen-antibody complexes and T cell products may enable the macrophage to present antigen to B cells in such a form as to trigger those cells for antibody production.

Macrophages may also function by **concentrating antigen** in 'critical sites', such as the follicles and medulla of the lymph nodes, thereby optimizing the chances of contact with lymphocytes. A further possibility is suggested by recent work indicating that macrophages can release 'soluble factors' (referred to as lymphocyte-activating factor or interleukin I) that can influence the activity of lymphocytes. The relative importance of these various macrophage activities in antibody production remains to be determined.

Some antigen may be retained at the surface of macrophages where it serves as a **depot of antigen** for the maintenance of the immune response. It is also possible that some antigen retained within the macrophage will function in this way although antigen can also be **catabolised** within the macrophage and later eliminated from the body as breakdown products. Macrophages have receptors for the Fc component of immunoglobulin and for C3b (p. 23). These will enable complexes of antibody and antigen to adhere to the macrophage membrane and be subsequently internalised.

Immune tolerance
Another possible result of the interaction of certain types of antigen, e.g. soluble protein antigens, with the surface of lymphocytes

is that the cell is prevented in some way from transforming for antibody production and is thus functionally eliminated from further participation in the immune response. This phenomenon is known as **immune tolerance** and is specific for the inducing antigen, and the term is used by immunologists to indicate a state in which the individual is unable to respond to a specific antigen or hapten. The phenomenon was recognised in 1924 by Glenny and Hopkins. Owen in 1945 observed that dizygotic cattle twins parabiosed in utero by placental fusion were permanent chimeras with respect to their red cells. Immune tolerance was first studied experimentally by Medawar and his colleagues in mice injected neonatally with cells from another strain of mice (i.e. containing transplantation antigens) (p. 161). The injected mice were later able to accept grafts from the strain of mice which had donated the original injected cells.

It has since been found that tolerance to a large variety of antigens can be readily induced when the antigens are injected neonatally. Tolerance can also be induced in the adult provided more antigen is given to take into account the maturity of the lymphoid system, the larger size of the lymphoid organs and more cells to paralyse. A notable advance was made in this field when Mitchison, using serum protein antigens, showed that there was another form of tolerance inducible by very small doses of antigen. This was termed **low zone tolerance** in contrast to the high zone tolerance previously described. Doses between these two levels were found to immunise. Other workers have confirmed these findings with different types of antigen.

Tolerance induced in either the T cell or B cell populations of lymphocytes results (as would be predicted from what is known of co-operation between the two cell populations) in tolerance of the whole animal to the antigen used to induce tolerance. This was established by transferring either tolerant T cells or tolerant B cells to a recipient mouse that had been irradiated and injected with normal cells of one or other population (i.e. T or B cells). Tolerant T cells would not co-operate with normal B cells to produce an immune response to human gammaglobulin and tolerant B cells would not co-operate with normal T cells to produce a response. The T cell population appeared to retain their tolerance for rather longer than the B cells (approximately 150 days compared to 50 days).

An additional complication has recently been noted by the finding that there appear to be two T cell populations. One cooperates with B cells to produce an immune response; the other

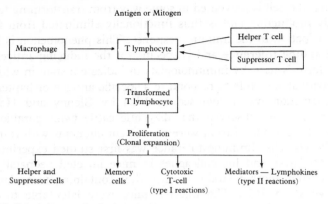

Fig. 4.19 T lymphocytes in the immune response

appears to be able to inhibit or suppress B cells. **Suppressor T cells** seem to act early in the immune response and may be involved in the early stages of tolerance induction. They may act by recognising the idiotypic determinants (p. 69) of the surface immunoglobulins of B cells and could be responsible for maintaining self-tolerance by suppressing those B cells expressing anti self immunoglobulin receptors.

Figure 4.19 summarizes the interrelationships between T lymphocytes and macrophages leading to development of helper and suppressor T cells and clonal expansion of T cell populations. The immunity provided by cytotoxic T cells is often referred to as type I reactions and the immunity derived from the production of soluble mediators as type II reactions.

Immunoglobulin synthesis
After the initial changes of transformation of lymphocytes have been set in motion, the actual **synthesis** of large amounts of immunoglobulin takes place. Two types of cell have been shown to be engaged in this process: (1) cells of the **plasmocytic** series and (2) cells of the **lymphocytic** series (small, medium and large lymphocytes). Of these two types the plasma cell line makes the largest contribution to immunoglobulin production and when single cells from immunised animals are examined in microdrops it can be shown that two-thirds of the **antibody-producing cells** are of this type (Fig. 4.20). An important characteristic of any cell making immunoglobulin is the presence of a **rough endoplasmic reticulum** (formed by the attachment of protein-synthesising polyribosomes to the convoluted endoplasmic reticulum membrane). The lympho-

Endoplasmic reticulum
with attached ribosomal
(RNA) granules

Antibody secretion
(Russell body)

Mitochondrion

Golgi apparatus

Nucleus

Nucleolus

Fig. 4.20 Plasma cell

cytes contain less of this than do plasma cells. It has been shown by a number of techniques that the immunoglobulin is localised in the spaces of the endoplasmic reticulum where it sometimes forms distinct aggregates termed Russell bodies.

In the spleen the cells engaged in antibody production tend to be found in the **red pulp**, and in the lymph glands in the **cortex**.

Individual immunoglobulin-producing cells appear to be able to synthesise the whole molecule, both heavy and light polypeptide chains (p. 67). It has also been found that the individual cells make only one class of immunoglobulin and that the light chains are restricted to only one of the two types (K and L, p. 67). It is very unusual to find an immunoglobulin secreting cell synthesising more than one class of immunoglobulin, although B cells in the early stages of an immune response can be shown to be secreting IgM antibody. They later switch to the synthesis of IgG antibody and thus at any one time produce only one class of immunoglobulin. Recent evidence indicates that the same cell can switch back to IgM production during a secondary response. The IgG that is produced is of the same specificity as the earlier IgM and almost certainly involves continued synthesis of the same light chain and the same variable region of the heavy chain; only the constant region is altered. The genetic mechanism may be a translocation event whereby the variable region gene becomes dissociated from the μ constant region gene and associates with the γ constant region gene. This IgM-IgG switch seems very likely to depend upon the influence of T cells on the B cell population.

The actual synthesis of immunoglobulin (after DNA has directed the synthesis of the appropriate mRNA) is carried out on the ribosomes of the producing cell, tRNAs sequentially adding amino acids to the growing polypeptide chain. Different ribosomes synthesise heavy and light chains, and assembly (by disulphide bond formation) takes place after the chains have been released into the cisternae of the endoplasmic reticulum. Polymerization of immunoglobulin molecules to form IgM involves the addition of J chains and carbohydrate groups just prior to its release from the cell.

Monoclonal antibodies

A very important advance in the rapidly expanding field of biotechnology comes from the development by Milstein and Kohler in Cambridge of 'immortal' cell lines capable of producing antibody of any required specificity, indefinitely, in cell culture conditions.

In conventional immunisation procedures injection of purified antigen leads to the production of an antiserum containing antibodies with a wide range of specificities for different determinants on the antigen molecule. It is virtually impossible to separate the different antibodies to obtain those of a particular specificity. The technique used to produce monoclonal antibodies does not require the preparation of purified antigen for injection and enables the selection of a cell producing antibody of a single specificity that is then grown in bulk to produce large amounts of the specific antibody.

The principle behind the method is the fusing of cells from an immunised animal with cells of a cultured myeloma cell line. Polyethylene glycol is the agent used to fuse the two types of cell. The myeloma cells are selected for their ability to grow in 8-azaguanine because they lack the enzyme hypoxanthine guanine phosphoribosyl transferase. This enzyme is required for rapid growth in tissue culture medium containing hypoxanthine, aminopterin and thymidine (HAT medium).

After fusion, the cells are grown in HAT medium in a number of wells for 10–14 days. The supernatants of each well are then tested for antibody activity. Clones that secrete the required antibodies, usually only a small proportion of the cultures, are selected and grown in bulk. This can be done either in culture or as tumours in the peritoneal cavity of mice; the antibodies are secreted into the tissue culture fluid or the peritoneal fluid of the mice. The technique is outlined in Figure 4.21.

The potential value of the technique is vast and will enable the identification of differentiation antigens on cells, cell receptors,

Mouse injected with antigen
↓
Spleen cells removed
↓
Fused to myeloma cells
↓
Hybrids grown in HAT medium
in wells
↓
Supernatants tested for required
antibody
↓
Clones secreting required
antibody selected and grown
in bulk

Fig. 4.21 Production of moloclonal antibodies

tumour antigens, histocompatibility antigens, microorganisms and their products or tissue cells. New applications are appearing continually and radioimmunoassay techniques, tissue typing and serotyping of microorganisms will be revolutionised within the next few years. The regulation of the immune response by such antibodies is not inconceivable and the passive use of monoclonal antibodies to treat infections or tumours is within the bounds of possibility. The use of antibody to D antigen of the rhesus system (see p. 153) to prevent haemolytic disease of the newborn will be of immediate value and anti-idiotypic (p. 209) autoantibody potentially could suppress autoantibody formation.

The development of monoclonal antibodies from human cells has been achieved by work in Scotland utilising a modification of the original technique so that the myeloma cell line is chemically treated before fusion and only cells that fuse are able to survive.

The extension of the technique to cell-mediated immunity is now under way using activated T lymphocytes fused with lymphoma cells. Such hybridomas offer the possibility of enhancing suppressor or helper cell activity to particular antigens and could have wide application in the future.

Gut-associated lymphoid tissue and antibody production
The thymus appears to control the cells of the cell-mediated immune system (p. 90) probably by providing facilities for the maturation of immature bone marrow cells. The cells of the immune system concerned with producing circulating antibodies reside mainly in the cortico-medullary junction and medullary cords of lymph nodes and the red pulp of the spleen.

The search for an equivalent of the bursa in mammals, including man, is not yet complete but the evidence suggests that the fetal liver is the primary site of B cell development and that the bone marrow takes over later (see p. 48).

THE CELLULAR PROCESSES
INVOLVED IN ANTIBODY FORMATION

Learning and memory. The outstanding feature underlying these mechanisms is that the immune response is a **learning process** at the cellular level.

After initial contact with an antigen the cells of the immune system retain a memory which can be evoked on subsequent contact with the antigen, and furthermore, like other learning processes, the immune system becomes increasingly skilled with continued experience of a particular antigen. The antibody which is synthesised becomes increasingly more effective in binding with antigens, as those cells which are best able to produce a 'good fitting' (avid) antibody molecule are selected from the population of antibody-forming cells. At the same time increasing numbers of committed cells are added to the immune system on repeated contact with antigen and the magnitude of the response is increased (p. 59). This increase in quantity and **avidity** of antibody can lead for example to increased efficiency in neutralising an infective agent or its toxic products so that a well-immunised animal would be able to withstand a dose of the agent which might be lethal to a poorly immunised animal.

The immunological memory can exist for the lifetime of an individual and implies that memory T and B cells are long-lived. Some of these cells are likely to be non-dividing and others divide at a low frequency. The intermitotic intervals can extend from a few months in rodents to at least 10 years in man.

Theories of antibody production

Two main theories have evolved which account for antibody synthesis and are referred to as **directive** and **selective** theories.

Directive theory. The **directive** theory was formulated by Haurowitz, Mudd and Alexander in the early 1930s and later modified by Pauling. The antigen is visualised as a mould or template which can enter any immunoglobulin-producing cell and cause the pattern of amino acids laid down to be modified so that it will fit the template, resulting in the synthesis of a molecule with a spatial configuration complementary to that of the antigen molecule. To account for the continued production of antibody it is assumed that the antigen, or part of it, remains in the cell to direct future antibody production. Alternatively, it is proposed that the antigen modifies the genetic information in the DNA of the cell so that it and its daughter cells continue to produce the specific immunoglobulin.

Selective theory. In contrast, the **selective** theory proposes that antigen selects, from the population of cells capable of making antibody, only those few cells that already have the inherent ability to make an immunoglobulin specific for the antigen. The antigen serves simply as a trigger on reacting with antibody receptor sites at the lymphocyte cell membrane. The **clonal selection theory** of Burnet is the best known of the selective theories and was formulated and modified over the years to take account of the hitherto unexplained phenomenon of recognition by the normal individual of tissue antigens as part of self and distinguishing these from foreign non-self antigens. Such an explanation became necessary with the description of human diseases where self-recognition breaks down and self antigen is treated as if it were foreign antigen — so-called autoimmune disease (p. 201). The theory proposes that the cells of the antibody-forming system have arisen by random mutation resulting in the emergence of small numbers of cells or clones of cells differentiated so as to be capable of producing one or a very small number of specific antibodies. Contact by such differentiated cells with self or foreign antigenic material during fetal life before the cells have reached maturity, would lead to suppression rather than stimulation of antibody formation against the particular antigen concerned — **immune tolerance**. That this could occur was illustrated by Medawar and his colleagues. Mice could be induced to accept potentially incompatible skin grafts by pretreatment during neonatal life with the appropriate 'transplantation antigen'. These studies were the forerunner of much further work in this field and it has now been shown that tolerance can also be induced even in adult animals if antigen is given in suitable doses and in an appropriate manner. However, it is more difficult to do this in the adult, the immature immune system of the neonatal animal being more susceptible. X-irradiation of an adult is frequently used as an aid in tolerance induction (p. 168).

Burnet has since suggested that the initial contact with self antigens leading to the elimination of 'self-reactive clones' or 'forbidden clones', may take place in the thymus, this organ acting as a **censor** of the lymphoid cells. This idea is supported by the very rapid turnover of lymphocytes in that organ and by the emergence of self-reactive antibody-producing cells in the absence of the thymus. The view is held by some immunologists that the ageing process may in part be due to a failure in these proposed controlling mechanisms, i.e. a gradual loss of efficiency of the censorship role of the thymus associated with its atrophy later in life.

The immune response to an antigen and the consequences of repeated stimulation can readily be explained in terms of the selective theory.

Antigen introduced into an animal comes in contact with lymphocytes carrying receptors corresponding to the antigenic determinants of the antigen molecule (p. 76). Some receptors (high affinity receptors) will fit the determinant well whilst others (low affinity receptors) will not fit so well. The dose of antigen given will have an effect on whether more antigen is bound by high or low affinity receptors — the less antigen given, the greater the chance that cells with high affinity receptors will bind antigen. With increasing doses of antigen more will be available to combine with the lymphocytes with the weaker lower affinity receptors. The consequence of this is that large doses of antigen will generate antibody of low average affinity and small doses will generate high affinity antibody. On subsequent administration of antigen, antibodies of progressively **higher affinity** will be produced. This is because after the first dose of antigen its concentration will gradually fall in the tissues as it is gradually catabolised and eliminated, resulting in less antigen being available for the lymphocytes with low affinity receptors. In these circumstances, lymphocytes with high affinity receptors will preferentially bind the small amounts of antigen remaining and will consequently be stimulated to produce high affinity antibody. This 'selection' of lymphocytes will be reflected in the **affinity** of the antibody stimulated by subsequent doses of antigen given to the immunised animal.

Implications and variations of theories. The theory outlined above suggests that early contact with self antigens leads to the individual developing an immune system which is suppressed or tolerant towards self antigens. The unblocking of a cell inherently capable of producing antibody against self antigen would explain **autoantibody** formation (p. 201). It is for this aspect of immunity in particular that the clonal selection theory provides a more plausible explanation than the directive theory which requires that all antibody-forming cells are blocked by every self antigen rather than only those cells capable of responding specifically to each antigen concerned. The other main characteristics of antibody formation — the specificity of antibody for antigen and the differences between the primary and secondary responses — can be explained equally well by either theory; the clonal selection theory is however the most complete attempt so far to take into account all the known facts of antibody production.

A number of variations of Burnet's original selective hypothesis have been proposed in the last few years but all maintain the assumption that the cell is already programmed to produce a specific antibody. It has been postulated, for example, that each potentially immunologically competent cell carries chromosomal DNA genes for a large variety of different types of antibody and is thus capable of responding to many antigens (sometimes referred to as the 'germ line theory'). An alternative proposal is that all antibody-producing cells may initially make identical immunoglobulins. During the lifetime of the individual variability of amino acid sequence appears due to crossing over during mitosis of the nucleotides responsible for coding the **variable** amino acid sequences of the Fab portion of the molecule. There is a clear survival value in such a variation-producing mechanism resulting in the production of immunoglobulins capable of reacting with a wide range of environmental antigens. Similarly there is survival value in the maintenance of those parts of the gene carrying the nucleotide sequences for the **constant** parts of the immunoglobulin molecule which maintain its structural integrity.

In conclusion, immunologists have yet to resolve the question as to whether the wide range of antibody specificity found in the adult animal is the result of **somatic mutation** within the lymphocyte population or whether the necessary information is encoded in the inherited **germ line** cells. Work by Milstein and his colleagues at Cambridge, using cultures of clones of mouse myeloma cell lines, showed some cells producing immunoglobulin which varied from that produced by other cells of the same clone. This suggests that somatic mutation had occurred in the structural genes coding for immunoglobulin heavy chains. This evidence is further supported by workers in Australia who removed single antibody-forming cells from a clone of cells and showed that in some cases their progeny were producing slightly different antibody. Evidence obtained by measuring the rate at which labelled messenger RNA or labelled DNA anneals with single stranded DNA from the parent genome indicates that there are probably only a small number of genes coding for the variable regions of the immunoglobulin molecule.

Work in the last few years has clearly demonstrated that somatic mutation occurs in the variable portions of both the heavy and light chains. It therefore seems that a large proportion of the variability in antibody molecules is caused by somatic mutation. The mutational process is not confined to the hypervariable regions but often occurs in other areas of the variable region. The process seems to be one that changes individual bases with occasional changes in two adjacent bases. The number of mutations in any one protein is so high that it is supposed that there must be a specific mechanism operating to increase the mutation rate. The evidence from variations between the V regions of early IgM antibody and later IgG and IgA antibodies make it likely that somatic mutation occurs after a given B lymphocyte encounters an antigen to which its surface immunoglobulin can bind. Thus somatic mutation will occur in the peripheral B lymphocyte population and would be followed by selection for B lymphocytes that express higher avidity antibody on their surface.

This would argue strongly for somatic mutations making an important contribution to antibody diversity. Recent work suggests a mechanism that appears to contribute to germ line diversity, involving an 'insertion sequence' carried in the germ line cells. This segment of DNA has identical ends and is inserted between the front end of the V region and the joining region at its tail. This allows the V region to proliferate by repeated gene duplications independently of its tail.

Both the theories, germ line and somatic mutation, are thus combined to make a contribution to antibody diversity. Further diversity may be generated by mutations and reduplications at the tail component, the J region. This can lead to the possibility of many V regions joining up to other J regions with resulting diversity of DNA sequences. The details of the molecular events involved in these processes are beyond the scope of this introductory text and the reader should refer to advanced articles listed under 'Further Reading' for details.

The idea that an antigen selects and reacts with a pre-existing lymphocyte receptor specific for the antigenic determinant should not be interpreted too strictly. It is inconceivable that each individual carries an infinite number of lymphocytes with appropriate receptors for an infinite number of antigenic determinants. Remembering that the combining site of an antibody molecule recognises the shape of an antigenic determinant (p. 33) then one combining site will be able to recognise two or more antigenic determinants with very similar (although not identical) shapes (Fig. 4.22). It has been estimated that a minimum of $10^4 - 10^5$ antibody combining sites (existing as receptors on lymphocytes) are required to provide the 'shapes' necessary to combine with all possible antigenic determinants.

THE CELL-MEDIATED ACQUIRED IMMUNE RESPONSE

In the immunologically mature individual, contact with an antigen leads not only to the production of circulating antibody, but also to the development of a separate cell-mediated form of response. In both types initial contact with the antigen is necessary and the response is specific for the antigen. Cell-mediated immunity occurs particularly in infections by agents which enter the cells such as

Fig. 4.22 Diagrammatic view of combining ability of an antibody molecule directed primarily at antigenic determinant A but able to combine also (cross-react) with antigenic determinant B. The strength of the bond will be less when the antibody is combined with determinant B as the molecules will be in less close apposition.

viruses, tubercle bacilli and *Brucella* species (p. 121). It can also develop after skin contact with certain simple chemical substances (p. 194). The sequence of steps leading to this form of immunity is essentially no different from that leading to the antibody response but the response is initiated in different areas of the spleen and lymph nodes (white pulp around the central arterioles of the spleen and the paracortical areas of the lymph nodes); these areas are under the control of the thymus gland (p. 42).

A characteristic of these thymus-dependent lymphocytes is that they can be stimulated to differentiate and divide by plant extracts known as phytohaemagglutinins (PHA) and by certain extracts of microorganisms such as streptolysin S from streptococci. These substances, sometimes referred to as mitogens, appear to act on the small lymphocytes of all vertebrates so far examined and induce enlargement of the cells, increased synthesis of RNA followed later by DNA synthesis. The plant extracts are specific for sugar determinants present in the lymphocyte cell membrane, and interaction leads to 'triggering' of the activity of the cell. This involves biochemical changes that are now beginning to be understood and include transport of ions (e.g. Ca^{2+}), amino acids and nucleotides through the cell membrane leading to purine synthesis and finally cell division. This process is known as **lymphocyte transformation** and can be brought about in sensitised lymphocytes on subsequent expo-

Table 4.5   Main steps in lymphocyte transformation

1.	Reaction of inducer at plasma membrane — PHA or antigen
2.	Increased synthesis of RNA in 30 min to 2 hours
3. Morphological changes —	enlargement of the cell, changes in nucleus,
(transformation)	increases in lysosome granules and endocytosis
	(commences at about 20 hours)
4.	Increase in thymidine incorporation into DNA about 36 hours for PHA and 40 hours for antigens. Mitosis

sure to the sensitising antigen. (See Table 4.5.) Transformation is readily measured in vitro by culturing the cells in the presence of labelled precursors of nucleic acids, e.g. ^{14}C thymidine for DNA synthesis or ^{14}C uridine for RNA synthesis. The test can be used to detect sensitisation to an antigen and the non-specific plant mitogens are used as a test of the competence of the cell-mediated immune system. Lymphocytes from an individual with, for example, an immune deficiency state (Ch. 5) with thymic aplasia and consequent defective cell-mediated immunity would be unable to transform in the presence of PHA. Transformation of lymphocytes to PHA is reduced in certain virus infections (p. 128).

Mechanisms of cell-mediated immunity

Lymphocyte activation products
Cell-mediated immunity dependent on these activated lymphocytes is usually recognised by means of a skin test (e.g. intradermal injection) with the antigen that, in an individual who has developed a cell-mediated immune response, results in an inflammatory reaction at the injection site. When examined histologically it can be seen that the tissues at the injection site have been infiltrated by mononuclear cells, mainly lymphocytes and a few macrophages. There is considerable experimental evidence that the majority of the infiltrating cells are not the activated (or sensitized) lymphocytes that have previously been sensitised to antigen but uncommitted cells attracted by soluble products of the sensitised lymphocytes.

Lymphokines. These are soluble products of activated lymphocytes (sometimes called lymphocyte activation products — LAPs) produced by exposure of sensitised lymphocytes to the sensitising antigen. They are believed to serve three main functions: (1) **recruitment** of uncommitted lymphocytes, (2) **retention** of such cells and phagocytes at the inflammatory site and (3) **activation** of the retained cells so that they can take part in the inflammatory response. These products can be thought of as chemical messengers that allow **communication** between the cells and also as agents that **amplify** the response. They act on macrophages, polymorphs, lymphocytes and also on other non-lymphoid cells.

The best known of these non-antibody factors released by sensitised lymphocytes on contact with antigen has the property of preventing the in vitro migration of macrophages on a glass surface. Macrophages can be set up in culture in small capillary tubes and will normally migrate out of the open end of the tube into the culture fluid (Fig. 4.23). A factor released from lymphocytes exposed to antigen will prevent this migration by causing the macrophages to stick together. This factor is likely to be released also in vivo and may be responsible for the accumulation of macrophages in cell-mediated immune reactions (p. 122). Purification and identification of those factors are very difficult as they are produced in very small amounts. Guinea pig macrophage inhibitory factor appears to be a glycoprotein with a molecular weight of 35–50 000, but its mechanism of action is unknown. Another, probably different, factor that affects macrophages has the property of activating the cells.

Small culture chamber

Horizontal glass cover slip

Tissue culture fluid with—NO ANTIGEN

Macrophage migration from tube

Piece of capillary tube containing peritoneal exudate cells (macrophages and a few lymphocytes)

Tissue culture fluid WITH ADDED ANTIGEN

No migration of macrophages

Fig. 4.23 Macrophage migration inhibition test

Such activated macrophages can be shown to have increased bactericidal activity as well as activity against tumour cells (p. 178).

A further as yet undefined factor released from sensitised lymphocytes after exposure to antigen causes stimulation and proliferation of normal unsensitised lymphocytes. This is known as mitogenic factor. Yet another lymphokine has a chemotactic effect on macrophages attracting them to the site of the inflammatory response. A cytotoxic effect, which appears to be due to a lymphokine (lymphotoxin), has also been demonstrated with a damaging effect on a variety of types of cell. A factor which increases capillary permeability (skin reactive factor) can also be shown to be released by sensitised lymphocytes. A number of as yet uncharacterised factors that appear to modulate antibody production by B cells have been described. Some are able to enhance B cell activity whilst others suppress antibody production.

The overall contribution of these factors in the cell-mediated immune response has not yet been clearly established, nor has their chemical identity or mode of action. However, it is widely believed that the lymphokines are the main effector mechanisms in the cell-mediated responses. When in vitro prepared lymphokines are injected into guinea-pig lymph nodes, lymphocytes accumulate in the paracortical region and there is enlargement of follicles with mitotic activation in germinal centres. A possible adjuvant effect is suggested for lymphokines as lymph node injection leads to an enhanced response to injected antigen. Lymphokines can be recovered in the afferent lymph in the primary immune response in a lymph node, from explants of granulomata in culture (e.g. schistosomia granulomata, p. 134), and in rheumatoid synovial fluids. Intradermal injection of lymphokines induces exudation of plasma proteins and inflammatory cells, and intraperitoneal injection aggregates macrophages in the intraperitoneal fluid exudate. Table 4.6 shows some of these lymphocyte activation products and the suggested in vivo activities of the factors.

In vivo role of cell-mediated immunity

It seems likely that the cell-mediated immune response is involved in protection against various infective agents (p. 126). It may also serve an important physiological role in the normal individual bringing about the elimination of spontaneously arising neoplastic cells which might represent a potential threat to the individual. In support of the existence of such an **immunological surveillance** mechanism (Ch. 8), it has been found that the incidence of tumours is highest at the two extremes of life when the immunological

Table 4.6

Lymphokine activity	Possible role in vivo
Macrophage 'migration inhibition'	Retention of emigrated macrophages at site of inflammation
Macrophage 'chemotaxis'	Emigration of macrophages to site of inflammation
Macrophage 'activation'	Enhanced metabolic, phagocytic and antimicrobial activities
Macrophage 'aggregation'	Aggregation and localisation of macrophages at inflammatory site.
Macrophage 'arming'	Enhanced extracellular cytotoxic effects of macrophages
Macrophage 'spreading-inhibition'	Brings about cell surface changes possibly facilitating passage of cells through blood vessel walls
Lymphocyte 'mitogenesis'	Induces non-committed lymphocytes to become metabolically active at inflammatory site
Lymphocyte 'potentiation'	Augmentation of lymphocyte activation by specific antigen
Lymphocyte 'suppression'	Limitation of DNA synthesis by lymphocytes
Lymphocyte 'co-operation'	Facilitation of B cell response to T-dependent antigens
Granulocyte 'migration inhibition'	Similar effect as on macrophages
Granulocyte 'chemotaxis inhibition'	Similar effect as on macrophages
'Cytotoxic' effects	Induces lymphocyte cytotoxicity on certain cell types
'Inhibition of proliferation'	Inhibition of cell proliferation without lysis
'Virus suppression'	Interferon-like factors protecting from virus infection

mechanisms are at their least efficient. The cell-mediated immune system is under the influence of the thymus and the cells are referred to as thymus-dependent or T cells. After thymectomy in mice the incidence of tumours induced by chemical carcinogens and viruses has been found to be significantly higher than in sham-thymectomised controls. The thymus has been found to be absent in certain rare immune deficiency states of children (p. 199). In such conditions there is a deficiency of lymphocytes from the areas of spleen and lymph nodes under thymic control. Cell-mediated immune reactions are absent and there is an inability to deal with virus infections. This type of cell-mediated immune mechanism would be likely to have arisen **early in evolution** with the development of multicellular organisms and would have additional survival value in that it would also be effective against exogenous parasites.

Cellular traffic in other lymphoid tissues

In a previous section (p. 42) consideration was given to the traffic of lymphocytes from the bone marrow via the thymus to the lymph nodes. This journey, during which the cells are maturing and proliferating, probably takes a period of weeks. Another form of lymphocytic traffic also exists, involving a non-dividing population of small lymphocytes with a potential life-span of many months and derived mainly from the thymus. This journey is measured in hours rather than days (Fig. 4.24). This traffic takes the form of a **recirculation** of small lymphocytes between the blood and lymphoid tissue, and thus each small lymphocyte may be exchanged between these two compartments very many times during its lifetime. One of the main advantages to the individual of such a recirculation process is that, for example, during the course of a natural infection the continual traffic of lymphocytes would enable very many different lymphocytes to have **access to the antigen** with the result that there would be a good chance that a lymphocyte carrying antibody receptor for the particular antigen would come across it and initiate an immune reaction. Another possible role of this recirculation process is that it can be used to **replenish** the lymphoid tissue of, for example, the spleen which might have been depleted by X-irradiation, trauma or infection.

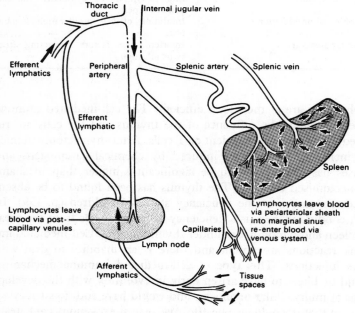

Fig. 4.24 Schematic view of main pathways of lymphocyte circulation

There is convincing evidence that lymphoid tissues can **recruit** lymphocytes from the recirculating pool. If a rat spleen is irradiated immediately after an intravenous injection of sheep red cells the antibody response is only slightly delayed. However, if whole-body irradiation is given after the initial splenic irradiation there is complete suppression of the anti-sheep cell response. It thus seems likely that without whole-body irradiation the irradiated spleen is able to recruit a fresh supply of lymphocytes from the circulating pool.

Another situation in which recirculation of lymphocytes could be helpful in the induction of an immune response is when the local concentration of antigen might be sufficient to induce tolerance rather than immunity in a static cell population. The passage of lymphocytes through an area where antigen had been localised and concentrated on the dendritic processes of macrophages might facilitate the induction of immunity.

The routes of lymphocyte recirculation

There are three main areas where the migration or transfer of lymphocytes from the blood takes place: the **lymph nodes** and Peyer's patches, the **spleen** and the peripheral **blood vessels**. Most is known about the mechanism of transfer in the lymph nodes where studies using the electron microscope show that small lymphocytes actually penetrate and traverse the cytoplasm of the cuboidal endothelial cells of the post-capillary venules. These **post-capillary venules** are confined to the deep and mid zones of the lymph node cortex and are unusual in that their endothelial cells are hypertrophied and cuboidal in appearance in comparison with the flattened endothelium of normal post-capillary venules found elsewhere. From the lymph node cortex the lymphocytes pass through the node to the medullary sinuses and then to the efferent lymphatics.

The precise routes of lymphocyte migration in the peripheral blood circulation are not clear, but the migration seems to be on a much smaller scale than in lymphoid tissues and almost certainly takes place across capillary walls. The flow can be increased if a local granuloma is formed in response to some foreign agent; then the migration from blood to lymph can be as great as in the lymph nodes themselves.

In the spleen, post-capillary venules have not been described and it appears that small lymphocytes enter the periarteriolar sheath from the blood, passing between the cells rather than through them as in the post-capillary venules. The cells later re-enter the blood within the spleen rather than leave via the lymphatics.

Cell co-operation and the genetic control of the immune response

Despite the wealth of experimental data, the conclusions of which have been summarised in the preceding paragraphs, the precise mechanisms by which immunocompetent cells co-operate together to produce an immune response remains clouded in mystery. In the last few years new light, but by no means complete illumination, has been shed on the problem by the realisation that certain genes controlling the ability of the immunocompetent cells to respond to antigen are genetically very closely related to those genes controlling certain important cell surface antigens. These antigens are those involved in rejection of grafts and on transfer of a graft of tissue to an unrelated (allogeneic) recipient are recognised as foreign. An immune response is initiated and the graft is rejected (see p. 160).

The cell surface antigens are known as **histocompatibility** antigens and the group of genes that determines the expression of these antigens as the **major histocompatibility complex** (MHC). In the mouse these genes are present in chromosome number 17 and, as has been noted above, are closely related in this chromosome to the genes that control the immune response — referred to as the immune response (**Ir**) **genes or I region**.

Alloantisera obtained by immunisation between different mouse strains have identified two major regions, each defined by a major genetic locus. These are the K and D regions (see Fig. 4.25). They are important antigens in graft rejection, the first histocompatibility antigens to be recognised. The genes making up a given histocompatibility complex are termed a haplotype (see Ch. 7 for human histocompatibility antigens and their role in graft rejection).

H2-D and H2-K antigens are widely distributed in the tissues. All lymphoid cells express these antigens as do liver, lung and kidney cells and, to a lesser extent, brain and skeletal muscle. The K and D antigens are glycoproteins of molecular weight 43 000 associated with $\alpha 2$ microglobulins. These may, as noted earlier, have a common evolutionary origin along with immunoglobulin domains (p. 64). The K and D molecules show a variety of antigenic

Fig. 4.25 Major histocompatibility complex of the mouse

specificities sometimes unique for a given haplotype (private specificities) or sometimes shared between different haplotypes (public specificities).

The I region appears to determine certain surface antigens on T and B lymphocytes. Some of these antigens can be found on both T and B cells whilst others appear to be restricted to one cell type. T helper cells (see p. 43) and B cells appear to carry one of these antigens, whilst suppressor T cells (p. 78), only, carry another antigen. These I region determined surface antigens like the Ly antigens (p. 44) are likely to prove useful in subdividing lymphocyte cell populations with respect to their different functional activities.

The I region contains genes which function as lymphocyte activating determinants and code for membrane — associated antigens, the Ia antigens. Figure 4.25 shows the five subgroups so far determined within the I region. Various roles have been found for the different I regions in the immune response. Antisera against I region associated antigens block certain functions of the immune system, for example, the mixed lymphocyte reaction induced when genetically dissimilar lymphocytes are cultured together. Ia antigens are also concerned in T cell help and T cell suppression. The I–J region is associated with T cell suppression and cells carrying I–A and I–E determined antigens are involved in B cell help and delayed hypersensitivity reactions. The Ia antigens are surface glycoproteins composed of α and β chains of 33 000 and 28 000 molecular weight respectively. These antigens are expressed primarily on a proportion of B lymphocytes and macrophages and appear to play a crucial role in determining antigen presentation and T cell–B cell interactions. T cells detect antigen on the surfaces of antigen-presenting cells in association with Ia molecules and it is from this starting point that that the various immune regulatory events follow.

The first clues that the MHC genes were involved in cell co-operation came from studies on collaboration between thymocytes and bone marrow cells in the immune response to sheep red blood cells. It was found that allogeneic thymocytes and bone marrow cells collaborate poorly and that the most efficient response was produced when the cells were from syngeneic donors. Genetic analysis revealed that concordance in the I region of the mouse MHC genes was necessary for efficient collaboration. The same conclusions have more recently been drawn from studies of collaboration between macrophages and lymphocytes. These studies have important implications in immunity to infection, particularly in the case of virus infections, and are discussed more fully in Chapter 5 (p. 131).

The precise mechanisms underlying these effects are not clear but it is known that activation of T lymphocytes by antigen can be prevented by antisera directed against cell surface antigens controlled by the MHC genes. This suggested that the antisera were in some way blocking the receptor for antigen on T cells. Further studies have extended those observations and indicate that some gene product coded for by the MHC genes is involved in the steps that lead up to co-operation between T and B cells and possibly also in macrophage — T lymphocyte interactions. The nature of this gene product is not yet established, but recent work has indicated that in certain experimental systems in the mouse, a factor can be recovered from T lymphocytes that have been exposed to antigen (so-called educated T cells). This 'factor' can aid B lymphocytes in responses to certain antigens, and it seems possible that the factor may be the gene product involved in cell co-operation. The factor has been shown not to be an immunoglobulin and, significantly, is removed by antisera directed at MHC products. Immunologists await with interest identification of its chemical nature and the mechanism of its action on B lymphocytes.

The immunocyte complex
In this chapter the details of the origin of the immunoglobulins from lymphoid tissues and cells have been set out. The role of the thymus in influencing these cells has been described and an outline has been given of the traffic of lymphocytes between the various lymphoid organs. Details of the individual behaviour of particular cell population or tissues should not obscure the fact that the immune response is a highly complex process involving finely balanced **inter-relationships** between many different types of differentiated cell, e.g. macrophages, T lymphocytes, B lymphocytes, and influenced overall by the behaviour of the central lymphoid organs, e.g. the thymus and possibly other glandular tissues such as the pituitary.

The differentiated lymphoid cells involved in the immune response are all derived initially from the haemopoietic **stem cells** of the bone marrow. Bone marrow stem cells also differentiate to produce erythrocytes, thrombocytes, granulocytes and monocytes. The macrophages of the tissues and blood are derived from the latter cell. Figure 4.26 illustrates this schematically and shows the cells

Fig. 4.26 Differentation of bone marrow derived stem cells into blood elements and the immunocyte complex

that make up what is referred to as the 'immunocyte complex' consisting of T and B lymphocytes capable of responding to antigen and called **antigen sensitive cells** (or sometimes antigen reactive cells) and the cells which actually mediate the immune response and are actively committed to this; these cells are referred to as **immunocytes.**

The T and B lymphocytes of the immunocyte complex are seeded from the bone marrow stem cells via the primary lymphoid organs — the thymus and fetal liver (or the bone marrow in adults), and enter the secondary lymphoid tissues — the spleen, lymph nodes and the recirculating pool of the blood and lymphatics. The proportion of the different cell types in each of these areas varies somewhat, T lymphocytes predominating in the thymus and recirculating pool and B lymphocytes predominating in the bone marrow and spleen. Table 4.7 summarises this information and in addition provides details of the cell surface markers that characterise these cells, some of which are used to distinguish the two populations.

Table 4.7   Characteristics of T and B lymphocytes

	Percentage of cells (mice)	
	T lymphocytes	B lymphocytes
Location		
Peripheral blood lymphocytes	60–85%	25–35%
Lymph node cells	60–75%	25–35%
Splenic lymphocytes	25–45%	60–60%
Bone marrow cells	1–5%	35–45%
Thymus cells	> 95%	negligible
Thoracic duct cells	80–90%	10–20%
Markers		
Thy 1 antigen	present	absent
TL	present	absent
H–2 antigens	present	present
Ly antigen	present	present
	(Ly 1, 2, 3)	(Ly 5)
Immunoglobulin		
IgG or IgA or IgM	absent	present
or IgD or IgE		
Fc and C3 receptors	absent	present
	(usually)	

FURTHER READING

Baird A T (ed) 1975 Immunology, a scope monograph, 3rd edn. Upjohn, Michigan

Baltimore D 1981 Somatic mutation gains its place among the generators of diversity. Cell 26: 295

Barrett J T 1974 Textbook of immunology, 2nd edn. Kimpton, London

Bernacerraf B, Unanue E R 1979 Textbook of immunology. Williams and Wilkins, Baltimore

Bloom B R 1971 In vitro approaches to the mechanism of cell-mediated immune reactions. Advances in Immunology 13: 102

Burnet F M 1969 Cellular Immunity. Cambridge University Press

Cohen S, Milstein C 1967 Structure and biological properties of immunoglobulins. Advances in Immunology 7: 1

Cohen S, Humphrey J H, Coombs R R A 1967 Antibodies, structure and biological function. Proceedings of the Royal Society of Medicine 60: 589

Dresser D W, Mitchison N A 1968 The mechanism of immunological paralysis. Advances in Immunology 8: 129

Edelman G M 1970 The structure and function of antibodies. Scientific American 223: 34

Ford W L, Gowans J L 1969 The traffic of lymphocytes. Seminars in Haematology 6: 67

Fudenberg H H, Stites D P, Caldwell J L, Wells J V 1976 Basic and clinical immunology, 2nd edn. Lange, Los Altos

Hildemann W H, Clark E A, Raison R L 1981 Comprehensive immunogenetics. Blackwell, Oxford

Humphrey J H, White R G 1970 Immunology for students of medicine, 3rd edn. Blackwell, Oxford

Kabat E A 1968 Structural concepts in immunology and immunochemistry. Holt, Rinehart and Winston, New York

McConnell I, Monro A, Waldmann H 1981 The immune system. A course on the molecular and cellular basis of immunity, 2nd edn. Blackwell, Oxford

Marchalonis J J 1976 Comparative immunology. Blackwell, Oxford

Mitchison N A 1968 Immunological paralysis as a dosage phenomenon. In: Cinader B (ed) Regulation of the antibody response. Thomas, Springfield, III., p 54

Nelson D S (ed) 1976 Immunobiology of the macrophage. Academic Press, New York

Pick E, Turk J L 1972 The biological activities of soluble lymphocyte products. Clinical and Experimental Immunology 10: 1

Playfair J H L 1971 Cell cooperation in the immune response. Clinical and Experimental Immunology 8: 839

Playfair J H L 1979 Immunology at a glance. Blackwell, Oxford

Rogers Brambell F W 1970 The transmission of passive immunity from mother to young. North Holland, Amsterdam

Rosenthal A S 1975 Immune recognition. Academic Press, New York

Weiss L 1972 The cells and tissues of the immune system. Prentice-Hall, Englewood Cliffs, N.J.

Wolstenholme G E W, Knight J 1970 Hormones and the immune response. Ciba Foundation Study Group no. 36. Churchill, London

World Health Organisation 1976 Immunological adjuvants. WHO Technical report series no. 595

Note: Immunology Today, published monthly by Elsevier Biomedical Press, contains useful up to date review articles on basic immunology.

Immunology in Action

5

Infection, immunity and protection

Objectives
On completion of this section the reader will be able to:
1. Differentiate infection from disease
2. Define the compromised host syndrome and give three examples
3. List two common commensal organisms present on skin, in throat, nasopharynx, oropharynx, small intestine, large intestine, and female genital tract
4. List two ways in which the normal flora of the body prevents colonization and infection by pathogenic organisms and list two conditions by which this ecological balance can be disturbed
5. Give four examples of the mechanisms by which microorganisms can escape the immune response and establish themselves in the host's tissues
6. List three factors that contribute to 'nonspecific' immunity to microorganisms
7. Describe the role of immunological memory in the mechanisms of immunity to bacterial and viral infections
8. Define antigenic drift
9. Give three examples of bacteria and viruses that depress cell-mediated immunity
10. List two factors associated with difficulty in development of an immune response to protozoa and helminths
11. Describe with the aid of a diagram the various consequences following stimulation of the T lymphocyte response to a microorganism
12. List three bacterial and three viral vaccines; describe their use in prophylaxis, and list any contraindications for their use.

In the normal healthy individual, despite popular belief, the relationship between microorganisms and ourselves is usually a harmless one. Saprophytic or commensal microorganisms grow and reproduce without apparent damage to either host or microbe. As

Lewis Thomas points out in his essay on 'Germs' (*The lives of a cell*, Bantam Books), 'we have always been a relatively minor interest of the vast microbial world' and human disease is not 'the work of an organised, modernised kind of demonology, in which bacteria are the most visible and centrally placed adversaries . . . . Most bacteria are totally preoccupied with browsing, altering the configurations of organic molecules so that they become usable for the energy needs of other forms of life.' The normal flora of humans is shown in Figures 5.1 to 5.3 and gives examples of bacteria, fungi and protozoa which are commensals. Parasitic microorganisms can very often be considered to be foolish commensals that do not recognise a good situation.

Modern medical science has managed to eliminate many of the classical infectious diseases, but has also helped to create new ones which result from interference with normal host defence mechanisms — consequent upon medical and surgical procedures such as chemotherapy, catheterisation, immunosuppression and X-irradiation. Infections that develop in this way are known as iatrogenic (physician-induced) diseases in which host defence mechanisms have been **compromised** in some way (Table 5.1).

It is important to differentiate infection from disease. A host may be infected with a particular microorganism and be unaware of the presence of the microorganism. If the microbe reproduces itself to such an extent that toxic products or sheer numbers of organisms begin to harm the host then a disease process has developed. It is well known that certain viruses cause latent infections (e.g. Herpes simplex) and only cause disease (e.g. cold sores) under circumstances when the host defences are impaired. Other examples are the carriage of potentially pathogenic bacteria in the nose, throat or bowel, e.g. pneumococci, streptococci or salmonellae. This is known as the carrier state and is a source of infection to other individuals.

Evasion

Once a microorganism becomes established in the tissues, having escaped the innate defence mechanisms described in Chapter 2, the microorganism can often make use of a number of evasion strategies that protect it from the immune reactions of the host, including interference with phagocytic activity and antibody function.

For example, the pneumococcus secretes large quantities of capsular polysaccharide that repels phagocytes and mops up anti-

NOSE & NASAL PHARYNX

Staphylococci
Diphtheroids
Neisseria sp
Haemophilus sp

OROPHARYNX

Staphylococci
Streptococcus sp
Neisseria sp
Haemophilus sp

MOUTH

Staphylococci
Streptococci
Actinomyces sp
Haemophilus sp
Yeasts
Enteric bacteria
Anaerobic bacteria
Spirochaetes

SKIN

Staphylococci
Streptococci
Corynebacterium
Propionibacterium
Yeasts
Diphtheroids
Enteric bacteria (rare)

Fig. 5.1 Normal flora of the skin, mouth, nose and nasopharynx, and the oropharynx. (Reproduced from Blackwell CC, Weir DM 1981 Principles of infection and immunity in patient care. Churchill Livingstone, Edinburgh, p. 53)

GASTROINTESTINAL SYSTEM

STOMACH

Normally sterile

SMALL INTESTINE

Lactobacilli
Enterococci
Diphtheroids
Yeasts (<u>Candida</u>)   } Small numbers
Enteric bacteria
Anaerobic gram
negative bacilli

LARGE INTESTINE

Anaerobic bacteria
  gram negative
    <u>Bacteroides</u> spp
    <u>Fusobacterium</u> spp
  gram positive
    <u>Eubacterium</u> spp
    Lactobacilli
    <u>Clostridium</u> spp
    <u>Bifidobacterium</u>
    Streptococci

Facultative and aerobic organisms
  Staphylococci
  Enterococci
  Enteric bacteria
  <u>Proteus</u> spp
  <u>Pseudomonas</u> spp
  Yeasts (<u>Candida</u>)

Fig. 5.2 Normal flora of the gastrointestinal system. (Reproduced from Blackwell & Weir 1981, p. 54)

GENITOURINARY TRACT

KIDNEYS AND BLADDER

Normally sterile

VAGINA AND CERVIX

Anaerobic bacteria
  Lactobacilli
  Streptococci
  <u>Bacteroides</u> spp
  <u>Clostridium</u> spp
  <u>Bifidobacterium</u>
  <u>Eubacterium</u>

Aerobic bacteria
  Diphtheroids
  Staphylococci
  Enterococci
  <u>Strep. pyogenes</u> (group B)
  Enteric bacteria

Yeasts
  <u>Candida</u>
Protozoa
  <u>Trichomonas vaginalis</u>
  (10-15% normal women)

Fig. 5.3 Normal flora of the genitourinary tract. (Reproduced from Blackwell & Weir 1981, p. 55)

body as it is produced, thus allowing the pneumococcus itself to proliferate unhindered. Trypanosomes appear to change their surface antigenic make-up from one generation to the next, so that the antibody made in response to the antigens of the original organism is inactive against the second generation of organisms. Many microorganisms, particularly tubercle bacilli, brucellae and many viruses, disappear inside tissue cells before sufficient antibody is produced to act against them. In the last few years it has been found that leprosy bacilli, which are similar in many ways to tuber-

Table 5.1   The compromised host

Predisposing factor	Effect on Immune system	Type of infection
Drug or X-rays in immunosuppression Allograft recipients (renal, bone marrow, heart)	Diminished cell-mediated and humoral immunity	Lung infections, bacteraemia, fungal infections, urinary tract infections
Virus immunosuppression e.g. rubella, herpes, EB virus, hepatitis virus	Replication of virus in lymphoid cells with resulting impaired function	Secondary bacterial infections
Tumours	Replacement of cells of immune system	Bacteraemia, pneumonia, urinary tract infections
Malnutrition	Lymphoid hypoplasia Decrease in circulating lymphocytes Decreased phagocytic ability	Measles, tuberculosis, respiratory infections, gastrointestinal infections
Smoking, inhalation of dust particles (e.g. silica, fungal spores)	Inflammatory lung changes, immune complex deposition to fungal spores	Chronic respiratory infections, allergic responses
Chronic endocrine disease (e.g. diabetes)	Decreased phagocytic activity	Staph. infections Tuberculosis Respiratory infections, bacteraemia etc.
Primary immune deficiency (see Ch. 7)	Diminished cell-mediated and/or humoral immunity	

cle bacilli, have the ability to grow in the thymus-dependent areas of the lymphoid tissues. This affects the development of a cell-mediated immune response (p. 92) against the invading organisms and allows its unhindered proliferation. The same appears to be true for cutaneous leishmaniasis where instances have been described of a loss of cell-mediated immunity. In short, a particular microorganism is pathogenic because in some way it is able to circumvent, at least initially, the immune mechanisms of the host. Table 5.2 gives a list of microorganisms that have been shown to interfere with cell-mediated immune function. In a situation where the host immune defence mechanisms are defective in some way (often called the compromised host), the distinction between pathogenic and non-pathogenic microorganisms becomes unimportant. All microorganisms that are human parasites have the capacity to produce infection in such a defective host. The breakdown of the normal host-parasite relationship then assumes central importance.

Table 5.2 Microorganisms affecting cell mediated immune function

Bacteria	Viruses	Fungi
M. tuberculosis	Influenza	*Coccidioides*
M. leprae	Viral hepatitis	*Cryptococcus*
T. pallidum	Herpes simplex	*Histoplasma*
Brucella abortus	Cytomegalovirus	*Candida*
Salmonella spp.	Measles	
	Mumps	
	Rubella	
	Infectious mononucleosis	

Restoration of normal immune function is likely to be of more importance in the recovery of the patient than specific antimicrobial drug treatment.

Aggressins and impedins
These are a rather ill-defined group of bacterial products (Table 5.3), the presence of which is associated with virulence. If antibody to the aggressin is present the pathogenicity of the microorganism is likely to be reduced. They are usually enzymes and many have damaging effects on leucocyte function, for example leucocidins produced by many Gram-positive bacteria. *Staphylococcus aureus* produces at least three separate leucocidins acting on macrophages and polymorphonuclear leucocytes causing membrane disruption and degranulation. Injection of these substances into experimental animals can lead to leucopenia. The leucocidin diphosphopyridine nucleotidase acts within the phagocyte and destroys it. DNAases and nicotine adenine dinucleotidase have a similar effect. Other aggressins such as hyaluronidase act as spreading factors enabling dissemination of microorganisms through the tissues. Protein A from staphylococci combines with the Fc portion of the IgG im-

Table 5.3 Some examples of bacterial aggressins and 'impedins'

Staphylococci	Coagulase
	Leucocidins
	Hyaluronidase
	Protein A
Streptococci	Haemolysins
	Hyaluronidase
	Fibrinolysin
	Leucocidins
Neisseria gonorrhoea	IgA proteases
N. meningitidis	
Strept. sanguis	
Ps. aeruginosa	Collagenase
	Elastase

munoglobulin molecule (except IgG$_3$ subclass) and prevents complexes of antibody and antigen binding to the Fc receptor on phagocytes. This is an example of what is termed an **impedin** as are the IgA proteases produced by Neisseriae and certain streptococci (Table 5.3).

Epithelial attachment and infection

The attachment of a microorganism to an epithelial surface is a prerequisite for the development of an infectious process (excluding entry at sites of trauma). The mucosal surfaces of the respiratory, intestinal and genitourinary tracts are of primary importance as sites of attachment of microorganisms. Certain streptococci that are normal inhabitants of the mouth have been shown to adhere to epithelial cells of the cheek, whilst others preferentially attach to tooth surfaces. Specific attachment of various bacteria to different parts of the intestinal tract may account for the nature of the indigenous flora of the gut. It is suggested that the pathogenicity of *Salmonella typhi* and *Corynebacterium diphtheriae* depends on their ability to attach to the intestinal or pharyngeal mucosa respectively and *Neisseria gonorrhoeae* is believed to attach to epithelial cells of the genitourinary tract by means of its 'pili'. This organism at the

Table 5.4   Some examples of the ways in which microorganisms can sidetrack the immune mechanisms

Microorganism	Method of evasion
Pneumococcus	Capsular polysaccharide mops up antibody and prevents opsonization
Virulent strains of *Staph. aureus*	Anti-inflammatory factor limiting increased vascular permeability and access of antibody, complement and cells
Intracellular organisms (e.g. tubercle bacilli, brucellae, viruses, leprosy bacilli,	Intracellular localization prevents access of protective antibody
Certain viruses, e.g. rubella, herpes, Newcastle disease virus, hepatitis virus, murine leukaemia viruses, leprosy bacilli, leishmania organisms, malaria parasites	Interference with immune induction by effects on T lymphocytes or macrophages
Trypanosomes, malaria parasites	Immunosuppressive effects, antigenic variation in successive generations so that antibody is ineffective
Schistosomes	Antigenic disguise by incorporating host antigens in cell wall
Neisseria gonorrhoeae	Produces factor that breaks down IgA$_1$

same time appears to secrete an enzyme that breaks down secretory IgA_1, whilst IgA_2 is not affected. The portal of entry of microorganisms in a number of infective states is shown in Table 5.5.

Table 5.5 Portals of entry of microorganisms

Portal of entry	Infection
Ingestion	food poisoning, cholera, dysentery
Inhalation	measles, cold, flu
Sexual contact	gonorrhoea, syphilis, herpes virus
Iatrogenic	heart valves, pacemakers, wound infections
Zoonoses	malaria, salmonellosis, encephalitis, typhus
Self-infection	urinary tract, eye infection, appendicitis
Accidental	drug users, motor accidents

Infection and inflammation

The innate immune mechanisms that protect the individual (mechanical barriers, antibacterial substances and phagocytosis) have been discussed in Chapter 2 and this discussion is concerned with the protective responses that form a second line of defence. The microorganism, having successfully avoided the innate immune mechanisms, starts to proliferate in the tissues and its toxic products trigger an inflammatory response. The response is initiated by the release of vasoactive amines, principally histamine and SRS-A from mast cells. The resulting increase in vascular permeability leads to an exudation of serum proteins including components of complement, antibodies, blood clotting factors and phagocytic cells. Phagocytic cells are attracted to the site of inflammation by chemotactic factors generated by interaction of components of the complement system with antibody. C3a and C5a components are the chemotaxins. Anaphylatoxins generated at the same time increase vascular permeability and further encourage exudation of fluid and cells at the site of inflammation. See Chapter 2 (p. 19) for a more detailed discussion of the inflammatory response.

Many types of microorganisms (e.g. staphylococci, streptococci) are effectively dealt with by the polymorphs and the intensity and duration of the inflammatory process depends on the degree of success with which the microorganism initially established itself. This in turn depends on the extent of the injury, the amount of associated tissue damage and the number and type of microorganisms introduced. A localised abscess may arise at the site of infection.

Some capsulate microorganisms (e.g. pneumococci) are able to resist phagocytosis and are not dealt with effectively until large amounts of antibody are made. These mop up the released capsular polysaccharide and phagocytosis occurs. If bacteria are not eliminated at the site of entry and continue to proliferate, they may pass via the lymphatics to the regional lymph nodes causing their enlargement (lymphadenitis). Other microorganisms (e.g. diphtheria, tetanus, cholera) produce exotoxins and are called **toxigenic** organisms. In this situation they can produce their damaging effects without migrating from their site of entry. Immunity in this situation requires the development of specific **antitoxins** (see below).

The types of infection described above are usually referred to as **acute infections** and contrast with protracted or **chronic infection** which is usually induced by microorganisms that are adapted to live within the cells of the host. Included amongst these are mycobacterial infections (e.g. tuberculosis, leprosy) brucella infections and virus infections. In these infections cell-mediated immunity plays a predominant part in the final elimination of the microorganism.

IMMUNITY IN INFECTION

The immune system, as has been noted in Chapter 4, has evolved the capacity to respond and react to a large variety of foreign molecules whilst at the same time avoiding self-reactivity. The capacity of the individual to resist infection can be explained in terms of the clonal selection theory of acquired immunity with the production of a specific immune response. To understand the detailed cellular events and differences in responses to infection of individuals it is necessary to take into account more recently acquired knowledge of the role of the major histocompatibility complex (MHC) in determining the outcome of an immune response. The MHC is a highly polymorphic system of genes that control the expression of cell surface molecules involved in immunity (see p. 98).

The existence of such a polymorphic system will inevitably result in individuals with different immunological potentials to respond to a given challenge. Whilst some individuals will be well prepared to resist an infectious agent others will be at risk. It will come as no surprise to find that certain infective states are linked with the MHC. For example, the association between viral hepatitis and the HLA-A8 antigen on lymphocytes (see p. 210). There are many examples of such associations in viral infections of mice.

The evolutionary advantage to a species of such a polymorphic set of determinants of immunity, with its attendant survival value and possibility of adaptation, is clearly an advantage in dealing with unforeseen challenges.

Association between certain infections and the blood group status of the individual has also been established. Individuals of blood group O are more susceptible than those of other blood groups to cholera. There is also an increased susceptibility if they do not secrete blood group substances into their tissue fluids and mucous secretions (i.e. are non-secretors). Carriers of streptococci tend to be non-secretors. In studies of a Chilean population it was found that people of blood group B had a 50% greater probability than non-B persons of contracting *E. coli* urinary tract infections. Blood group B individuals are more susceptible to Neisseria infections. Non-B persons and non-secretors are more susceptible to rheumatic fever and rheumatic heart disease. In the author's laboratory, blood group B and AB non-secretors have been found to be 3 times more susceptible to urinary tract infections.

Bacterial infection

Antibody-mediated immunity

Antitoxins. Many microorganisms owe their pathogenic abilities to the production of **exotoxins**. Amongst diseases dependent on this type of mechanism are diphtheria, cholera, tetanus, gas gangrene and botulism.

Diphtheria toxin, for example, is a polypeptide chain with a molecular weight of about 62 000 daltons. The intact molecule is not active but requires the reduction of one disulphide bridge and hydrolysis of the peptide chain to release an active fragment. This is believed to occur at the membrane of host cells resulting in the entry of the toxic fragment into the cell where it interferes with protein synthesis. The cholera toxin owes its effects to its ability to bind to a specific glycolipid of the intestinal cell wall. A toxin constituent then passes through the cell wall, enters the cytoplasm and irreversibly 'switches on' the adenyl cyclase (the cyclic AMP-making enzyme). The 'activated' cell then proceeds to secrete fluid into the intestinal lumen resulting in massive fluid loss from the tissues.

Antibodies either acquired by immunisation or previous infection, or given passively as antiserum, are able to **neutralise** bacterial toxins. To give protection, antibodies must either be present in sufficient quantity, as they would after administration of antiserum, or be produced faster than the toxin is produced by the microorganism. This would be likely to occur if the individual had previously been exposed to the organism or its products by natural infection or artificial immunisation. In such a situation the infected

Fig. 5.4 Scheme showing the progress of infection and the immunological defence mechanisms

individual would be able to mount a rapid secondary immune response (p. 59). The previously exposed individual can be said to have an **immunological memory** of the toxin, having a population of cells ready and waiting to respond rapidly to the slightest whiff of the exotoxin. The infected individual with no 'immunological memory' may require to be given antibody prophylactically in order to tide him over the first stages of infection.

Bacterial toxins have been largely identified as enzymatic in nature and the antibody in some way is able to interfere with the ability of the enzyme to interact with its substrate. The antibody is not thought to interact with the active site of the enzyme but the nearer it reacts to this the more effective is its neutralising power likely to be. The most probable explanation of the inhibitory effect of antibody is that it produces what is called 'steric hindrance', which simply means that it gets in the way and physically prevents the enzyme from coming in close apposition to its substrate (Fig. 5.5). This idea is supported by the finding that antibody is much more effective against enzymes which have high molecular weight substrates than it is against those with low molecular weight substrates. Figure 5.5 shows how such a low molecular weight substrate can still come in contact with the active site of the enzyme even in the presence of antibody.

Enzyme molecule
Active site

Antibody molecule

Low molecular weight substrate

High molecular weight substrate

Fig. 5.5 Diagrammatic view of the possible 'steric hindrance' effect of antibody against an enzyme toxin. A low molecular weight substrate avoids the blocking effect of the antibody molecule. The closer the antibody is attached to the active site of the enzyme the more effective will be its blocking action

Antibacterial immunity. In the case of a microorganism that does not secrete exotoxins, the protection afforded by antibodies depends on the direct effect of antibodies attached to the surface of the microorganism. This can have a number of effects, the most important of which is in encouraging phagocytosis by macrophages of the blood (monocytes) or the polymorphonuclear leucocytes. Phagocytic cells have receptors for a site on the Fc fragment of immunoglobulin G (particularly the human IgG 1 and IgG 3 subclasses) that is exposed after the immunoglobulin has combined with its antigen. There are also receptors for the C3b component of complement. This means that a bacterium coated with antibody and complement will adhere to a phagocytic cell and become susceptible to phagocytosis (see also p. 17). The phagocytic cell in many instances can then digest the microorganism by secreting into the phagocytic vacuole a variety of digestive enzymes carried in the intracellular lysosomes. However, some microorganisms such as the streptococci and *Mycobacterium tuberculosis* are able to resist intracellular digestion. The streptococcus carries, as part of its cell wall, a substance known as M protein, which confers the ability to resist digestion by the enzymes. If immunity exists to the M protein, by previous exposure or artificial immunisation, the streptococcus is susceptible to intracellular digestion. Rough (avirulent) strains of salmonellae are susceptible to intracellular digestion whilst the smooth (virulent) strains are able to resist digestion in some way. In the case of enteric infections such as those due to *Salmonella typhi* or *Vibrio cholerae*, antibodies can be secreted into the intestinal lumen and attack the organism before it invades the intestinal mucosa. These antibodies secreted by an immune individual are known as copro-antibodies and are predominantly IgA. The IgA immunoglobulin is selectively produced in intestinal and respiratory mucous membranes (p. 74).

IgA can be detected in many mucous secretions in higher concentrations than found in serum, and IgA-producing plasma cells are found more commonly in the lamina propria of mucous membranes than in the spleen and lymph nodes. Various functions have been attributed to such IgA, and there is evidence that it acts as an antitoxin together with IgG in protection against experimental cholera infection. Another suggested function of IgA is that by reacting with gut microorganisms it prevents their adherence to the gut wall. This is suggested by experiments in mice in which cholera organisms were prevented from adhering to the gut wall by the presence of IgA. A further function of IgA is suggested by work with IgA fractions of human colostrum, which bind to *E. coli* together with complement. The effect of this on the lipopolysaccharide of the bacterial cell wall is postulated to lead to the exposure of the underlying mucopeptide. This enables the enzyme lysozyme (p. 15) to digest the mucopeptide layer with resulting lysis of the bacterium. Gram negative organisms such as *E. coli* are normally resistant to the effects of lysozyme (Fig. 5.6). It should be noted that these effects have been shown by in vitro assays and may not reflect what occurs in the intact animal. Other effects of antibody

Fig. 5.6 Gram negative bacillus showing lipopolysaccharide which protects mucopeptide cell wall from the effects of the mucolytic enzyme lysozyme. IgA + complement may attack the lipopolysaccharide and allow access of lysozyme to the cell wall

reacting with the surface of the microorganism are cell lysis, brought about by the activation of the complement system, and simple localisation of the organism by agglutination or clumping.

It is even conceivable that antibody acts by coating growing bacteria so that their daughter cells, when formed, remain in a clump instead of dispersing. Attachment of bacteria to the host's red blood cells in the presence of antibody and complement is another way in which phagocytosis is encouraged. This phenomenon is known as **immune adherence** but as yet it is not clear exactly how the attachment to red cells takes place.

Apart from the clumping effect on the bacteria, agglutination seems to have little effect on the viability or respiratory activity of the organisms, although it is conceivable that the bacteria at the centre of a large mass of clumped organisms would be limited in their metabolic activity simply by a lack of sufficient nutrient material. Recent work suggest that antibody can inhibit the uptake of iron by some bacteria and that its lack can inhibit their growth.

A possible protective role for IgE has been suggested by the finding of a similar distribution of this immunoglobulin to that found for IgA in the mucous secretions produced by local plasma cells. IgE is known to attach to the surface of mast cells and on combination with antigen, degranulation of the mast cell occurs with histamine release. These reactions in the allergic individual lead to hypersensitivity states (p. 181). If it occurs on a smaller scale in a localised area it might be helpful in bringing about an inflammatory response with consequent elimination of a microorganism.

Acquired cellular immunity

Macrophage-dependent cellular immunity (See Fig. 5.7). The interrelations of antibody-mediated immune mechanisms and acquired cellular immunity are not yet clearly defined. It is known, however, that macrophages from animals immune to tubercle bacilli are more actively phagocytic than those taken from a normal animal. The cells spread out more than unstimulated macrophages when cultured in a glass chamber, and are more heavily endowed with mitochondria and lysosomes. The cellular immunity fades with time but can be recalled in an accelerated manner only by exposure to the original antigenic stimulus. Enhancement of cellular immunity has been reported with macrophages from brucella-infected animals; such cells restricted the intracellular growth of brucellae although the enhancement was dependent on the initial immunisation with a living virulent strain of the organism. The same phe-

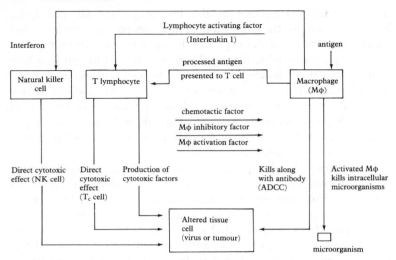

Fig. 5.7 T lymphocyte – macrophage relationships

nomenon has been found after *Listeria monocytogenes* infection in mice in which macrophages isolated from the peritoneal cavity acquire an increased resistance to listeria and at the same time an increased intracellular resistance to tubercle bacilli and brucellae. This increased resistance is **non-specific** in the immunological sense in that the enhanced activity of the macrophage is directed not only at the species of organism responsible for the initial infection but also at other species (see Table 4.6).

The non-specific enhancement of macrophage activity, including their ability to kill microorganisms and spread themselves throughout the peritoneal cavity to mop up an infectious agent, appears to depend partly upon the transfer of an as yet undefined stimulus from lymphoid cells which have reacted immunologically to the initial injection of microorganisms. Thus the first part of the response depends on a specific immune reaction on the part of lymphoid cells to an agent such as *L. monocytogenes*; these cells proliferate and in turn activate the macrophages so that not only do they handle listeria more effectively but also other bacterial agents. This phenomenon can be shown quite clearly by transferring stimulated mouse lymphoid cells to an unstimulated recipient; the recipient's macrophages then assume these enhanced bactericidal and spreading properties. These points emphasise that cellular immunity, though non-specific in its expression, is specific in its elicitation and that the non-specific component is a property of the macrophage and the specific component dependent on the lymphocyte.

Immunity in virus infections

Antibody-mediated immunity

Virus infections, particularly those caused by enteroviruses, are frequent and severe when humoral immunity is impaired as in inherited immunodeficiency states. In Bruton type deficiencies (see p. 197) poliomyelitis may develop after vaccination; meningoencephalitis caused by echovirus and coxsackie virus may also be seen. In a variety of mouse experimental models the administration of immunosuppressive drugs has shown that antibody is essential for recovery from a number of virus infections, including influenza and coxsackie viruses. Antibody appears to operate through opsonisation followed by ingestion by macrophages or by neutralisation of virus haemagglutinins.

In many situations viruses seem to be able to escape these protective mechanisms of the host and remain infective, even when complexed with antibody. Some viruses become latent, e.g. the herpes group, and are reactivated despite the presence of circulating antibody, passing from cell to cell without entering the bloodstream. Other escape mechanisms, such as that of the influenza virus, are discussed below.

Bloodstream or surface protection. In virus infections the efficiency of antibody depends largely on whether the virus passes through the bloodstream in order to reach its target organ. A well-known example of a virus which follows such a route is the **polio virus**; this crosses the intestinal wall, enters the bloodstream and passes to the spinal cord and brain where it proliferates. Small amounts of antibody in the blood can **neutralise** the virus before it reaches its target cells in the nervous system. A number of other viruses behave in the same way and pass through the bloodstream on their way to their target organ; examples are the viruses of measles, mumps, rubella and chickenpox. Disease caused by these viruses is characterised by a **prolonged** incubation period.

In comparison, in another group of virus diseases with a **short** incubation period such as influenza and the common cold, the viruses do not pass through the bloodstream, as their target organ is their site of entry to the body, namely the respiratory mucous membranes. In this type of infection, even a high blood level of antibody will be relatively ineffective against these viruses in comparison with its effect on the blood-borne viruses. For this antibody to act on such respiratory viruses it must pass through the mucous membranes into the respiratory secretion. Examination of the antibody content of mucous secretion has shown that in contrast to the blood there is very little IgG antibody and often no IgM and it thus appears that the mucous membranes are not very permeable to antibodies of these classes. However, it has been found that the predominant immunoglobulin in these secretions is IgA manufactured by plasma cells in the lamina propria of the mucous membranes. IgA present in nasal secretions has been shown to be responsible for most of the neutralising activity against common cold viruses. One conclusion which can be drawn from this is that conventional immunisation methods designed to produce high blood levels of antibody are unlikely to be effective against viruses which attack the mucous membranes, and some effort is being directed at developing methods for stimulating local antibody production of IgA type in the mucous membranes themselves. An example of this is the intranasal administration of a live attenuated influenza virus which has been used extensively in the United States and the Soviet Union and is now available in Britain.

It is generally believed that the best way to achieve protection against a viral disease is to use a live virus vaccine and it is clear that natural infections of humans by influenza virus confers more complete and long-lasting protection than does vaccination. There is evidence that cytotoxic T lymphocytes may be as important as immunoglobulins in this protection. Inactivated influenza vaccines and subunit vaccines result in antibody production but are much less efficient in inducing cytotoxic T lymphocytes in mice. The neutralising antibodies generated in influenza infection are highly specific for the haemagglutinin of the infecting virus. In contrast, cytotoxic T lymphocytes appear not to discriminate between different type A influenza viruses. Thus for efficient long-term immunity live vaccines appear to be preferable to inactivated vaccines.

The high degree of immunity provided by the oral polio vaccine seems likely in part to be due to locally produced antibody in the gut neutralising the virus even before it reaches the bloodstream. The presence of IgA antibody against polio virus has recently been demonstrated in the faeces, in duodenal fluid and in saliva. In contrast, after injection of inactivated virus vaccine no such antibodies could be found. The nasopharyngeal antibodies have been shown to persist for at least 300 days which is consistent with the long-term protection which the oral vaccine affords. It is of some interest that the levels of IgA antipolio antibody were found to be lower in children who had their tonsils and adenoids removed. Furthermore, primary vaccination in such children produced lower levels of these specific antibodies than in children who had not had their tonsils removed.

Persistence of virus and 'antigenic drift'. One of the major differences between viral and bacterial immunity is that the former is usually of much longer duration and in many instances lifelong, e.g. in measles and mumps. An explanation of this may be that some virus remains within tissue cells and is protected from immune rejection. Occasionally some virus material is released and thus maintains a persisting level of immunity. The possibility exists that such virus antigen will combine with antibody resulting in the formation of **toxic complexes** with ensuing hypersensitivity of type 3 (p. 190). The existence of such a phenomenon could have considerable importance in the pathogenesis of some viral diseases.

In those virus infections in which repeated attacks occur, e.g. influenza and the common cold, fresh infection is due to different strains of the virus which are relatively insusceptible to the antibodies induced by previous infection by other strains. Evidence for a persisting immunity to virus comes from studies in the Faroe islands where successive measles epidemics were separated by intervals of 65 and 31 years. Only those who had not been previously infected developed the disease. Persistence of antibody can also be shown after virus and other infections, for example in Eskimos, 40 years after polio virus infection.

Influenza epidemics have occurred at 2 to 3 year intervals over the last 40 years amd type B virus outbreaks tend to alternate with type A epidemics. Type A virus is responsible for pandemic influenza infections. Type C influenza virus rarely, if ever, gives rise to epidemics and no variants have been reported since it was first isolated in 1950. The main viral antigen responsible for inducing immunity is the haemagglutinin (HA). It is sometimes called the 'V' antigen and is thought to be located on the spikes projecting from the viral envelope. Influenza viruses types A and B have different HA antigens and within these two types there are a number of distinct families with HA antigens which differ markedly from one another. Antigenic differences between HA antigens form the basis for classification of the viruses into families of the same type. Neuraminidase is also a surface antigen of influenza viruses and is responsible for the ability of the viruses to attach to tissue cells including red blood cells. This allows its laboratory detection in a haemagglutination test (see p. 229). In type A infection, the families A, A_0, A_1 and A_2 have appeared successively, and each in turn has dominated the epidemic history of influenza for periods of 10 to 15 years and is then displaced by later antigenic variants. It is believed that this 'antigen drift' from one virus family to another is one of progressive mutation, and that immunity against earlier strains becomes obsolete once further antigenic variants have appeared. The consequence of antigenic drift is that new strains do not react well with antisera against older strains, although older strains tend to react well with antibody against the new strain. Antigenic drift is probably due to selective pressures brought about by antibody that favours the emergence of mutants supressing surface antigens sufficiently different as to be unable to combine with existing antibody.

There is a danger that mutants responsible for 'antigen drift' may emerge and dominate as a result of widespread use of vaccination procedures directed against strains responsible for epidemics. In this situation such insusceptible mutants would be 'selected' from the virus population and replace the previously dominant strain.

The phenomenon of 'antigen drift' is not limited to influenza virus and the argument outlined above has been used for not instituting nationwide vaccination as a means of protecting cattle from foot and mouth disease virus. The same difficulties stand in the way of the development of common cold vaccines.

Cell-mediated immunity

Virus elimination and tissue damage. The humoral immune response is probably the predominant form of immunity responsible for protection from reinfection by viruses. For this reason immunisation procedures aim at producing circulating or mucous membrane antibody. In the case of primary virus infections the position is not very clear but it seems likely to involve some form of cell-mediated immunity. It is known that children with congenital hypogammaglobulinaemia (p. 195) can recover from virus infections without producing any virus-neutralising antibody. Although it is possible that these children are producing small amounts of neutralising antibody sufficient to provide immunity, it is significant that the capacity to resist virus infection is associated with normal cell-mediated immune reactions. These subjects are able to develop normal delayed hypersensitivity reactions to bacterial and viral antigens and contact sensitivity to simple chemicals (p. 194). In patients with Swiss-type agammaglobulinaemia (p. 199), who have an additional cell-mediated immune deficiency, susceptibility to virus infection is very great and death often follows the development of severe generalised vaccinia after routine inoculation of live smallpox vaccine.

A laboratory model is available that has enabled the detailed study of the role of cell-mediated immunity in virus infection. Adult mice infected with lymphocytic choriomeningitis virus (LCM virus), which itself is not damaging to cells (non-cytopathic), develop clinical signs (e.g. meningitis) with the onset of an immune response to the virus. If this response is prevented by means of immunosuppressive agents (e.g. anti-lymphocyte serum, cytotoxic drugs, irradiation or thymectomy) then the disease does not develop. If an infected animal treated in this way is then given spleen cells from an untreated virus-infected animal, the pathological changes characteristic of the disease develop in the recipient. These changes are likely to be brought about by a cytotoxic factor (p. 95) released from the transferred spleen cells interacting with infected cells of the recipient. The consequences of this immune response can thus be seen to be twofold: (1) virus-infected cells are destroyed by stimulated spleen cells with the likely elimination of the virus; (2) host cells are themselves damaged and this is responsible for the pathological manifestations of the disease. Whether or not the pathological changes in any human virus infections depend on mechanisms of this type is not clear at present. However, some in vitro experiments in which cells infected with measles or mumps virus are destroyed by incubation with spleen cells of a virus-immunised animal suggest that such phenomena may take place in the disease state itself. Much additional work will be required before the picture becomes clear.

Further evidence that cell-mediated immune reactions are involved in resistance to viruses comes from the finding that, just as in the case of intracellular bacterial agents such as tubercle bacilli and brucellae, cell-mediated reactions of the delayed hypersensitivity type (p. 192) can be demonstrated after many types of virus infection. The best known example of this is the reaction soon after revaccination with vaccinia virus where there is an accelerated reaction (compared to primary vaccination) reaching its maximum at 72 hours with a minimum of tissue damage and a rapid elimination of the infective agent.

An important component of the cell-mediated response is the role of helper T lymphocytes that cooperate with macrophages and B lymphocytes for an optimal antibody response (see Fig. 5.7). Thymectomised animals show an impaired antibody response during virus infection with consequent reduced ability to eliminate virus.

Babies with congenital rubella infection have been shown to excrete virus for periods up to 18 months of age. Such infants can be shown to possess high levels of IgM anti-rubella antibody, which indicates that they have not developed neonatal tolerance (p. 87) to the virus. Their cell-mediated immune mechanisms seem, however, to be defective due to a direct effect of the virus on lymphocytes. Lymphocytes taken from such an infant do not respond normally to the plant mitogen PHA (p. 92) and normal leucocytes infected in vitro with the virus can be shown to become defective in the same way. **Depression of lymphocyte reactivity** has been associated with a number of virus infections, e.g. rubella, herpes, Newcastle disease virus (causing fowl pest) and hepatitis virus. Certain viruses are able to **replicate** in **macrophages** (e.g. arboviruses, murine hepatitis virus, lactate dehydrogenase virus and herpes simplex virus) and others do so in **lymphocytes** (e.g. lymphocytic choriomeningitis virus, leukaemia viruses and Epstein-Barr virus).

The effects on the activity of the immune system brought about by viral infection have been mainly studied with murine leukaemia viruses. Infection of mice with these viruses usually results in depression of the activity of the immune system affecting both humoral and cell-mediated immunity. In some instances (e.g. Friend virus infection) there is selective depression of a particular class of immunoglobulin (IgG) suggesting an effect on particular populations of lymphocytes. Graft rejection was found to be profoundly depressed in animals infected with gross leukaemia virus.

The mechanisms underlying these effects are not clear. Amongst the proposed mechanisms are: virus-induced changes in the **uptake** and processing of antigens; **destruction** of cells of the immune systems; antigenic **competition** by the virus preventing the host response to other antigens.

The clinical implications include: persistence of virus in the absence of a protective immune response; the development of immune complex disease (p. 190); potentiation of tumour growth as a result of depressed immunological capacity and thus of immune surveillance mechanisms (p. 174).

Recent studies have indicated that the lesions associated with virus infections cannot be explained simply by the cytopathic effects of the virus on cells. The immune response of the host to the viral antigen appears to play a role in producing tissue damage due to the immune complexes (see p. 190), formed by virus and antibody.

Cytotoxic T lymphocytes (Fig. 5.7) will kill histocompatible target cells (see p. 99) infected with a variety of viruses, e.g. LCM and influenza. Another protective mechanism operates through Fc receptor expressing cells such as macrophages that will lyse antibody treated virus infected cells. This is called anitbody dependent

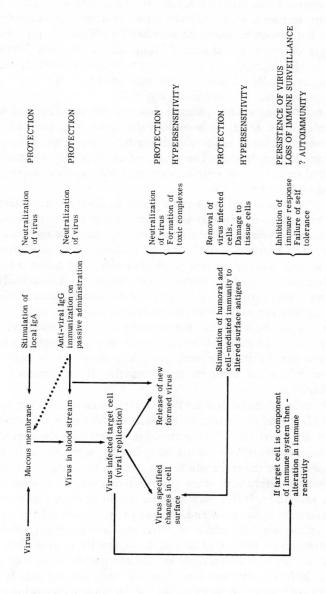

Fig. 5.8 Schematic view of virus infection and immune response, indicating some possible consequences

cell-mediated cytotoxicity (ADCC) (Fig. 5.7). The mechanism has been shown to be effective against mumps, herpes simplex, vaccinia, and influenza virus infected cells. Another lymphocyte population that cannot be identified as either T or B cells by their surface markers are the so-called natural killer cells or NK cells. These can destroy cells infected with a number of viruses — Epstein-Barr, coxsackie, and LCM viruses — and this ability of NK cells seems to be potentiated by interferon (Fig. 5.7).

If macrophages are rendered inactive by injections of silica, herpes simplex infections have been shown to be potentiated. Macrophages can restrict replication of hepatitis virus in the mouse; this is genetically controlled. The ability of macrophage cultures to resist viral replication in vitro is correlated with in vivo susceptibility or resistance to the virus.

Another way in which a virus can initiate destruction of host cells is by virus-induced changes in the surface antigens of the host cell. The altered surface antigen stimulates an immune response with subsequent destruction of the cell by antibody and complement and possible concomitant release of pharmacologically active mediators of inflammation (p. 183). Such a phenomenon is not necessarily detrimental only to the host cells as these are virus-infected cells and their elimination would lead also to destruction of the virus. In conclusion it can be seen that the outcome of a virus infection is the result of the **interplay** between **protective** and **hypersensitivity** mechanisms the balance usually settling in favour of protection. Figure 5.8 is an attempt to summarise these complex interrelationships.

Interferon. A quite distinct type of resistance mechanism in virus infection is the production by the infected host cells of a substance known as 'interferon'. This material interferes with the synthesis of new virus by tissue cells of the host. Interferon, unlike antibody, is not specific for the virus which may have induced its formation but is able to interfere with other quite different species of virus. Interferon probably plays a very important role in eliminating virus in non-immune individuals and the rise in level of interferon appears to coincide with the phase of virus elimination whilst circulating antibody levels are found to rise subsequently to this. The three types that have been described are summarised in Table 5.6.

The human interferon gene has now been synthesised. It is the largest gene so far synthesised in the laboratory consisting of 514 nucleotides. Genetic engineering methods will enable the gene, after insertion into an *E. coli* plasmid, to produce the substance in large quantities.

Table 5.6 Types of interferon

Type	Name	Source
α	leukocyte interferon	leukocyte buffy coats
β	fibroblast interferon	diploid fibroblastoid cultures
γ	immune interferon	T cell macrophage supernatants

Susceptibility to virus infections and the role of the major histocompatibility antigens in cellular response

In Chapter 4 consideration has been given to the genetic control of the immune response by a specific group of genes called **Ir genes**. These have been shown to be closely related to those genes controlling the major antigenic determinants of graft rejection (MHC genes). The possibility that a gene product closely associated with the MHC genes is involved in co-operation between T and B lymphocytes leading to an immune response is noted on page 99. This phenomenon is of interest in view of the known relationship between histocompatibility antigens (determined by the MHC gene complex) and susceptibility to certain virus-induced leukaemias in mice. The susceptibility of mice to lymphocytic-choriomeningitis virus (p. 127) may also be determined in this way. With increased knowledge of the gene complex controlling histocompatibility antigens and various functions of lymphocytes associated with the immune response, it should be possible in the next few years to elucidate some of the factors that determine susceptibility to virus diseases.

The role of the MHC in graft rejection was the first evidence that the control of the immune response depended on activities of the genes in that area (see p. 161).

It later became apparent that T and B lymphocyte interaction and macrophage T lymphocyte cooperation also required compatibility between the MHC regions of the cell types involved. In this instance surface molecules (Ia antigens) determined by I region genes are those involved and thus are important determinants of immunity to (1) intracellular bacterial infections and (2) in recognition of cellular interactions in antibody production. The H-2K and H-2D regions control surface molecules involved in cytotoxic T lymphocyte (Tc) (type 1) activities and thus determine protective immune responses to viruses as well as graft rejection (Fig. 4.25).

Since viruses can infect a large variety of different cell types the ubiquitous distribution of H-2K and H-2D antigens enable Tc cells to deal with virus infections of all cell types. In contrast Ia antigens are more limited in distribution, being found on cells of the immune system including a proportion of macrophages and on T and B lymphocytes. In view of their importance in generation of protective responses to intracellular bacteria they seem to act as receptors for signals leading to activation of macrophages and on B cells as receptors for T cell generated signals for B cell differentiation such as switching on of Ig production and changes from IgM to IgG.

One of the reasons proposed to explain why classical tropical parasites seem to generate rather poor immune responses is that they infect cells (e.g. malaria infecting red cells) outside the immune system and do not always lead to the expression of their antigen on the surface of the cell (in the way viruses do) and thus do not enable Tc cells to operate in a protective manner, although instances are being uncovered that suggest that at least some protozoal parasites appear to do so (see below). Their antigens are also not presented to the immune system in the way they would be if cells such as macrophages were infected.

Immunity to protozoa and helminths
The life cycles of organisms in this category are complicated and the immune response, to be effective, has to interrupt the cycle at a stage when the parasite is accessible to the immune processes.

Protozoa. Malaria infections are initiated by sporozoites which transform into exoerythrocytic schizonts in the liver, and at this stage there is recognisable immunity. The schizonts rupture and discharge their merozoites into the peripheral circulation where they invade erythrocytes. Antibodies are readily detectable in the serum and increase until the crisis 7 to 10 days later and then slowly decline. Because these antibodies are able to get access to the parasite only during a relatively short period of its life cycle, immunity is incomplete and the host usually fails to eliminate the parasite completely.

This state in which the organisms persist in small numbers in the tissues in the presence of an immune reaction is called **premunition** by parasitologists.

The IgG class of immunoglobulin is the major antibody class involved in acquired resistance to malaria and there is a considerable rise in the levels of, and rate of synthesis of, the IgG. However, if serum from an infected individual is incubated with parasitised erythrocytes, only a small quantity of the IgG antibody is absorbed. The major part of the IgG probably represents antibody to soluble malarial antigens, and seems unlikely to play a role in protection except perhaps when it is directed against toxic malarial products.

Parasitic growth within erythrocytes is unaffected by the presence of immune serum in the culture medium, but invasion of new red cells by merozoites and subsequent parasite multiplication is inhibited. IgG antibodies can bind to Fc receptors on macrophages (p. 19) and it seems likely that phagocytosis of antibody-coated merozoites is an important mechanism of acquired immunity. There is evidence that antibody may act on mature intraerythrocytic forms of the parasite, possibly due to expression of parasite antigen on the surface of the red cells that render the red cells susceptible to attack by antibody.

Considerable experimental evidence exists showing that malarial infection is associated with **immunosuppression** and that the extent of this parallels the degree of parasitaemia. It is not clear whether this has an effect on the immune response to the parasite itself. Depressed responsiveness of T lymphocytes to PHA (p. 92) and B lymphocytes to bacterial lipopolysaccharide can readily be demonstrated, as can diminished antibody responses to certain antigens. Further work will show the relative importance of cell-mediated and humoral immunity in malaria infections but at the moment humoral immunity appears to be the predominant protective mechanism.

The efficacy of the immune mechanisms against trypanosomes is complicated by the fact that the parasites can change their surface antigenic constitution from one generation to the next. The number of variants which can be produced by a single strain is at least 20. It is not yet clear how the organism controls the generation of the variants but variation is thought to arise by selection of mutants from a heterogeneous population of parasites.

This complication means that the immune response has great difficulty in keeping up with the antigenic changes in the parasite, and in the case of the trypanosomes responsible for African sleeping sickness, the parasite does not induce an effective immunity. The infected subject develops a progressive infection with invasion of the central nervous system leading to death. Trypanosomiasis is associated with high levels of IgM immunoglobulins in both the blood and CSF. It is not certain if this is due to the repeated new antigenic stimuli resulting from changes in the organism or if the parasite in some way influences directly the cells of the immune system. Increased immunoglobulin production is a common finding in protozoal infections and often affects all classes of immunoglobulins. Because usually less than 5% of the total immunoglobulin appears to react specifically with the inducing parasite, it is probable that protozoa stimulate the lymphoid cells in a non-specific way to overproduce immunoglobulins.

This type of evidence has turned the attention of immunologists away from a direct role for antibody in protection in protozoal infections towards antibody independent cell-mediated immunity. This, as has been noted, takes three forms: direct cytolysis by lymphocytes (Class I reactions), soluble lymphocyte products (Class II reactions) and natural killer cell (NK) activity. Recent evidence points to a central role for type 1 direct cytolytic reactions in an important tick-borne cattle disease, theileriosis, caused by several species of *Theileria* prevalent in several parts of Africa.

The lymphocyte-mediated cytotoxic reactions against infected cells have the same genetic restriction as virally infected cells in that the effector lymphocytes have to recognise both foreign and self MHC determined antigens simultaneously.

A similar phenomenon has been found in leishmaniasis and points the way to a better understanding of other protozoal infections including those of man.

An interesting example has recently been described of a protozoon that avoids elimination even in the presence of a vigorous immune response. *Entamoeba histolytica* exposed to fresh serum becomes markedly more resistant than untreated colonies to complement-mediated lysis. The effect appears to require active protein synthesis on the part of the protozoa suggesting a possible change in its membrane that resists the effect of activated complement components.

Helminths. Helminths, like protozoa, go through a complex life cycle and protective immune mechanisms appear to act only at an early stage in the cycle. The main stimulus appears to be due to antigens derived from the adult worm and the immunity derived from this acts on new parasites entering the body. A noteworthy feature of these infections is the appearance of IgE (reaginic) antibodies (p. 184) with pulmonary eosinophilia, and it seems likely that immediate hypersensitivity reactions of the anaphylactic type (type I) are involved in the pathogenesis of helminth infection. In *Schistosoma mansoni* infections the pathogenesis appears to be largely due to an **inflammatory granulomatous reaction** around the **schistosome eggs** trapped in the host tissues with a periovular area of necrosis surrounded by inflammatory cells, including many eosinophils. The most severe lesions occur during early infection. Mice in experimental schistosomiasis infections reject 70 to 80% of new infections 12 weeks after their first infection. In baboons a significant reduction in the damage done by the parasite to the host organs was found in pre-immunised animals. The experimental findings suggest a gradual waning of egg hypersensitivity but the mechanism is not understood. The tissues commonly affected are the liver, which shows chronic portal inflammation, the lungs, the kidneys and the spleen. The renal and splenic lesions are not directly related to the presence of worms or eggs, but may in part be due to immune complexes between worm antigens and antibody. In *Schistosoma haematobium* infection the urinary tract is the primary target and calcification of the bladder can occur in advanced cases. Migration of larvae into the lungs is sometimes associated with eosinophil infiltration and pneumonia which can be fatal.

These worms are believed to be able to protect themselves from host antibody by **incorporating host tissue antigens** in their cell wall. When worms are transferred from mice to monkeys that are immunised against mouse red blood cells, the worms are killed by an antibody-mediated reaction directed at the surface of the parasite. The host antigens acquired by the worms appear to be A, B and H blood group substances (p. 151) and possibly the Lewis antigen.

In many helminth infections there is an association between increased levels of eosinophils in the blood and high IgE levels. If eosinophils are experimentally depleted in mouse schistosome infections, immunity to the parasite is decreased. It is likely that lymphokines produced by T lymphocytes control the IgE and eosinophil response and that IgE on mast cells at the site of infection release mediators including chemotactic factor for eosinophils (ECFA). Eosinophils in conjunction with IgG adhere to the schistosomula and eosinophil enzymes destroy the parasite. Figure 5.9

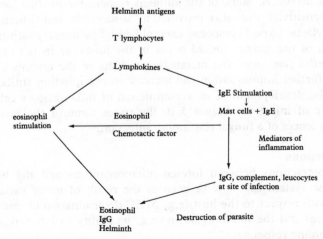

Fig. 5.9 Scheme showing the role of IgE and eosinophils in helminth immunity

illustrates the series of interactions involved. The eosinophil products include peroxidase and a basic protein, which are likely to be involved in the destruction of the parasite as well as enzymes that inactivate the mast cell products histamine and slow reacting substance of anaphylaxis (SRS-A) (see p. 183).

Saprophytic fungi and respiratory disease

Allergic alveolitis and anaphylaxis. A few examples of pulmonary hypersensitivity to inhaled fungal antigens have been reported in the last few years. The existence of a state of immunity has been confirmed by the finding of precipitating antibodies in the serum. The first of these disorders to be recognised was **farmers' lung** disease in which precipitating antibodies could be demonstrated against antigens derived from mouldy hay. The antigen has since been found to be *Micromonospora faeni*. Subsequently work in Edinburgh has demonstrated precipitins against *Aspergillus clavatus* in **maltworkers** exposed to high concentrations of *A. clavatus* spores from contaminated barley. Antibodies against *Coniosporum corticale* have been found in the serum of maple bark strippers.

It is likely that following exposure to high concentrations of any of a variety of fungal spores individuals would produce precipitating antibodies and thus this form of pulmonary hypersensitivity may be more widespread than has so far been identified. The hypersensitivity reaction induced by the presence of precipitating antibodies would be of the toxic-complex (type 3) form inducing a diffuse pulmonary interstitial pneumonitis which has been termed allergic alveolitis. Some of the antigens responsible for this form of hypersensitivity can also provoke in susceptible individuals the anaphylactic (type 1) response exemplified by pulmonary asthma. If growth of the fungus should occur in the lungs, as in the case of *Aspergillus fumigatus*, the metabolic products of the organism will cause further immunisation and increase in precipitating antibodies with the development of an accumulation of inflammatory cells at the site of infection. Figure 5.10 illustrates some of the possible consequences of a fungal respiratory infection.

Conclusions
The interactions between foreign microorganisms and the host's immune system can now be seen as the result of many variables both with respect to the host (e.g. MHC determination of immune response) and the microorganism (e.g. its ability to interfere with the immune response).

It is clear that the development of an acquired immune response

SPORES

TRACHEA

BRONCHI

IgA stimulation in mucous membrane
? protective

BRONCHIOLES

IgE stimulation
Type 1 anaphylaxis in walls of
air passages

ALVEOLAR DUCTS

Stimulation by fungi of serum
immunoglobulin
(detectable precipitating antibody)

IgG

Toxic-complex reactions
to inhaled spores

ALVEOLAR AIR SACS

Fungal antigens

Circulating toxic complexes
with fungal antigens

Possible growth of
organism (mycetoma)

Fig. 5.10 Scheme showing some of the possible consequences that may result from the inhalation of fungal spores

to a microorganism is no guarantee that the organism will be eliminated and that whilst often providing protection an immune response can sometimes be disadvantageous to the individual (e.g. immune complex production).

Figure 5.11 is an attempt to summarise the protective activities of the immune system with general application to the various types of microorganism discussed in this chapter.

Common vaccination procedures

Efficacy and hazards. It is generally accepted that one effective way of controlling the spread of infectious disease is by immunisa-

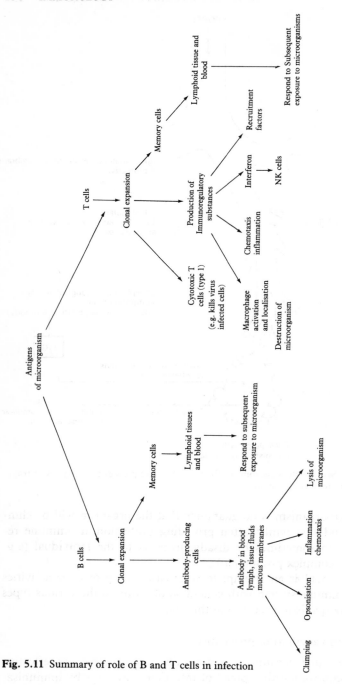

Fig. 5.11 Summary of role of B and T cells in infection

tion with antigens derived from the appropriate organism. The isolation and bulk preparation of the particular antigens which confer protective immunity is a major difficulty, but success in this field with a number of potentially dangerous microorganisms has radically altered the chances of them causing widespread disease in the population. The use of diphtheria toxoid (inactivated diphtheria toxin) is a noteworthy example. In Scotland, notifications of diphtheria averaged about 10 000 cases annually before 1940 when widespread immunisation was instituted. The incidence of the disease rapidly decreased thereafter and with the exception of an outbreak in 1968, involving six cases none of whom had been fully immunised, the disease can be said to have been virtually eradicated. Immunisation procedures are clearly not the only factor contributing to the decreasing morbidity and mortality from infectious disease. The combined death rate for scarlet fever, diphtheria, whooping cough and measles from 1860 to 1965 for children up to 15 years of age shows that nearly 90% of the total decline over the intervening century had occurred before widespread immunisation and the use of antibiotics. Improved environmental conditions and in particular, higher host-resistance due to improved nutrition, are probably major factors underlying the decline.

Much consideration has been given to the safety of vaccines and it is generally agreed that the greatest danger arises from the introduction of infection at the time of administration of the vacccine. Complications such as encephalitis after smallpox vaccination, febrile convulsions after whooping-cough vaccination and neurological complication after rabies vaccination are extremely rare phenomena. The risk is by far outweighed by the protection that immunisation can give from the disease itself.

Recombinant DNA techniques are likely to lead to the development of a variety of useful, widely available and inexpensive vaccines, including those for hepatitis B virus, typhoid and leprosy. Vaccination, rather than therapeutic intervention involving modification of immune regulation, seems a more hopeful approach to disease prevention, at least in the near future.

Immunisation of rhesus monkeys with a glucosyltransferase and purified protein antigens from *Streptococcus mutans* — the organism commonly associated with dental caries — results in protection from caries. The protective antibody appears to be IgG rather than IgA. It is hoped that after suitable safety trials this form of immunisation will prove useful in man in the prevention of caries with its widespread effect on dental health.

Antigens of microorganisms

Bacterial and viral antigens are in common use in medical practice as a means of inducing immunity to infectious diseases such as smallpox, diphtheria, measles, poliomyelitis, typhoid fever and many others. There are four main types of antigen preparations or **vaccines**.

1. **Toxoids** are the soluble exotoxins of bacteria, such as diphtheria and tetanus bacilli, which have been modified and rendered less toxic by the addition of formalin or gentle heating. They are administered either in solution or precipitated on alum. Many years of useful immunity can be achieved by these procedures.

2. **Killed vaccines** are cultured organisms killed by heat, usually 60°C for 1 hour, ultraviolet irradiation or chemicals such as phenol, alcohol or formalin. Protection against whooping cough, poliomyelitis and perhaps cholera can be achieved in this way.

3. **Antigens isolated from infectious agents**, for example the capsular polysaccharide of the pneumococci. A diffusable factor of *B. anthracis* and a cell wall preparation of haemolytic streptococci have been shown to induce immunity, but such preparations are not in general use in medical practice.

4. **Attenuated living vaccines** are made from strains of organisms that have lost their virulence by growth in culture (e.g. Pasteur's chicken cholera vaccine, p. 4) or in animals when the conditions are not favourable for the growth and proliferation of the virulent strain. Strains emerge which, whilst not able to produce disease, can induce immunity; such strains are known as **attenuated** organisms. The BCG vaccine (Bacille Calmette-Guérin) is the outstanding example of this type of vaccine, providing protection against tuberculosis in man. The oral administration of a strain of poliomyelitis virus induces a powerful immunity without producing the disease. The virus spreads from one individual to another and so is able to produce immunity in a community. An attenuated strain of yellow fever virus has been developed, obtained from the original virulent material by prolonged cultivation in tissue culture. Attenuated strains of measles virus are also used, and it seems likely that rubella virus vaccination will soon reduce the hazard of congenital abnormalities developing in the infants of mothers infected with the virus. See Table 5.7 for examples of common vaccines available for human infections.

In veterinary medicine successful vaccines have been produced against canine distemper, canine hepatitis and Newcastle disease (fowl pest) of chickens.

Table 5.7   Vaccine preparations in use in man

	Viral	Bacterial
A. Whole organisms Live (attennuated)	Smallpox Measles Rubella Polio Yellow fever Influenza (nasal vaccine)	B.C.G.
Inactivated (heat, UV, chemicals)	Influenza	Typhoid and paratyphoid
	Typhus	Pertussis Cholera
B. Products of organisms Toxoids		Diphtheria Tetanus

Routine procedures

The determining factors in the selection of immunisation procedures for a particular population must depend on local environmental conditions and epidemiological considerations. In Britain, a child is immunised during its first year of life with a vaccine containing diphtheria and tetanus toxoids in combination with a killed suspension of whooping-cough (*Bordetella pertussis*) organisms. This is known as **triple vaccine** and its efficacy as an immunising agent is in part due to the adjuvant effect of the pertussis component. This procedure is repeated on two further occasions and at the same time oral polio vaccine is usually given. Vaccination against smallpox is achieved by giving one dose of the vaccinia vaccine during the second year when the chances of developing complications appear to be much decreased. Primary vaccination is not advised after early childhood. The risk of serious complications in early childhood is very small but nevertheless considered to be out of proportion to the risk of being infected with the disease. Thus smallpox vaccination need no longer be recommended as a routine procedure in early childhood. Booster doses of all these vaccines are usually given at 5 years of age and tetanus, polio and smallpox again between the ages of 15 and 19. Table 5.8 shows the recommended schedules of the Department of Health and Social Security.

In the U.S.A. the official recommendation for childhood immunisation comprises the three primary doses of diph/tet/pert vaccine and oral polio vaccine at intervals of 4 to 6 weeks, beginning at the age of 2 to 3 months. A booster is given 1 year after completion of the primary course.

Live vaccines should not be given to persons whose ability to re-

Table 5.8 A schedule of vaccination immunisation procedures. After Joint Committee on vaccination and immunisation (1978)

Age	Vaccine	Interval	Notes
During first year of life 3 months	diph/tet/pert & oral polio vaccine* (first dose)		The first dose of triple vaccine together with oral polio vaccine should be given at 3 months. If pertussis vaccine is contraindicated or declined by parents diph/tet should be given
4½–5 months	polio vaccine* (second dose)	preferably after an interval of 6–8 weeks	
8½–11 months	diph/tet/pert & oral polio vaccine* (third dose)	preferably after an interval of 4–6 months	
During second year of life	measles*		
5 years of age or school entry	diph/tet/and oral polio*		
Between 11 and 13 years of age	BCG		for tuberculin-negative children
Girls between 11–13 years of age	rubella*		all girls this age should be offered rubella vaccine
Between 15–19 years of age or on leaving school	polio (oral* or inactivated tetanus)		whether or not there is a past history of the disease

* = live virus vaccines contraindicated during pregnancy.
(For full details and notes the reader should refer to Protection and Prevention 6th edition The Wellcome Medical Foundation Ltd., 1980).

spond to infection is reduced, as for example after radiotherapy, immunosuppressive drugs, steroids or in patients with immune-deficiency states. If a subject has had a local or general reaction to a vaccine, there is a risk of even more marked reactions to the next dose.

Special circumstances

Protective immunisation can be performed in situations where a particular hazard exists, such as to the fetus associated with rubella in pregnancy, the infectious hazards of travelling abroad, and the occupational hazards of acquiring certain infections. Table 5.9 shows situations when such immunisation procedures may be adopted.

Table 5.9   Disease against which protective immunisation may be provided in special circumstances

Hazards to the fetus Rubella	Hazards associated with occupation or other special circumstances
	Anthrax
Hazards to travellers	Influenza
Enteric fever	Mumps
Yellow fever	Plague
Cholera	Q fever
Smallpox	Rabies
	Tularaemia
	Typhus
	Hepatitis A & B (passive immunisation)

Immunisation against rubella

All girls should be immunised just before puberty with the live attenuated virus, regardless of whether they think that they have previously had rubella or not. This avoids the risk of their contracting the disease subsequently when they are pregnant, as rubella in pregnancy may lead to malformations of the fetus.

Female school teachers, nursery staff, and nurses and doctors caring for children in hospital and in clinics may be exposed to rubella; staff working in antenatal clinics may acquire the infection and pass it on to patients in the early stages of pregnancy. These groups should be offered rubella vaccination if preliminary serological tests are negative. However, as the vaccine should not be given during pregnancy, assurances must be sought from women in these groups that they are not pregnant and that they will take precautions against becoming pregnant for at least two months after taking the vaccine.

Immunisation of travellers

Travellers are exposed to infectious hazards that vary from country to country. There are national and international regulations which make vaccination against yellow fever, cholera and smallpox statutory for persons travelling to and from countries where the diseases are endemic, or where an epidemic has recently occurred. As the regulations are subject to change, a traveller who is visiting any country where the diseases have occurred in recent years should check from its embassy what certificates of vaccination are necessary, if any.

The traveller is often well advised to seek immunisation against other diseases that may be encountered (Table 5.9). Travellers may be unaware that poliomyelitis, diphtheria, tetanus and tuberculosis are still significant risks in some countries; medical students volunteering for work in developing countries should bear these special occupational hazards in mind. It is not yet possible to be artificially actively immunised against infectious hepatis (hepatitis A), but effective short-term passive protection is conferred by an injection of normal pooled human gamma globulin.

Occupational hazards

Immunisation against various infections considered above and also against mumps, Q fever, plague, tularaemia and typhus may be offered to laboratory workers and others at special risk.

In view of the success of the WHO smallpox eradication programme, vaccination against smallpox is no longer required as a routine in many countries. All doctors and nurses, and the staff of bacteriological laboratories and others who may meet previously unrecognised cases of smallpox or come into contact with infected material from them, should be revaccinated at least once every three years. This applies especially to the staff of hospitals for infectious diseases.

High titre hepatitis B immunoglobulin is available for the temporary passive protection of clinical and laboratory workers who sustain a skin-penetrating injury under circumstances associated with a risk of the transmission of the hepatitis B virus; prophylactic immunisation should soon become possible using antigens prepared in *E. coli* (p. 9).

An anthrax vaccine is recommended for those who handle animal hides and bones etc. Vaccination has similarly been practised against brucellosis and leptospirosis in man, but the protective value of available vaccines against these two occupational hazards is not established.

Notes on special vaccines

Enteric fever. TAB vaccine provides useful protection against typhoid fever, but its protective value against the paratyphoid fevers has not been proved. Tourists, business people and others who travel from countries in Northern and Western Europe and North America to Mediterranean countries, Africa, Asia and Latin America are advised to be immunised; this is obligatory for members of most armed forces. The paratyphoid components are omitted from **typhoid vaccine** and this is less likely to give the local and systemic reactions that are quite common with TAB vaccine.

Yellow fever vaccine. A preparation of live attenuated virus is given by injection and one dose confers immunity for 10 years.

Cholera vaccine. This vaccine is a preparation of killed cholera vibrios. Two subcutaneous injections with an interval of about 4–6 weeks give a degree of protection against *V. cholerae* and *V. eltor* that is unfortunately only transient.

Vaccination against smallpox. In the mid-1970s WHO announced that smallpox had been virtually eradicated, with only a few pockets of infection remaining in remote mountain villages of Ethiopia. By the end of 1976 Ethiopia seemed to be clear, but smallpox then occurred in Somalia, a non-endemic country which had been free of smallpox since 1963. The problem of the importation of this disease calls for a policy of 'ring vaccination' in which the contacts of any imported case are identified, located and vaccinated, and the population in these locations is offered prompt vaccination to contain the hazard. It follows that health workers who may have to deal at short notice with this emergency should continue to be vaccinated against smallpox, and doctors should know about smallpox vaccination which is given special consideration here.

Active immunity against smallpox is conferred by **vaccinia virus**; its origin is uncertain and it may be derived from variola or cowpox viruses. The vaccine consists of lymph obtained from vesicles produced on the skin of calves or sheep by inoculating the sacrified skin with the virus.

The vaccine lymph is supplied in glass capillary tubes or in plastic tubes (which are difficult to handle aseptically). If it is stored frozen, its potency is maintained for about a year at — 10°C and it may be kept in a domestic refrigerator for up to 2 weeks. It is inactivated at room temperature and no vaccine should be used after more than 7 days from the date of dispatch, unless it has been kept in a refrigerator. The vaccine is administered intradermally, usually on the upper arm, and the multiple pressure procedure is recommended. A drop of vaccine lymph is spread over an area of skin about 0.5 cm in diameter. The skin must be clean, but no disinfectant should be used. Pressure is applied to the skin through the vaccine with a sterile large flat needle, held so that it is almost parallel to the surface. To introduce the vaccine into the epidermis, the needle is applied quickly, but not so vigorously as to draw blood. From 10 to 30 such 'pressures' are recommended, ten sufficing usually for a 'take' in primary vaccination. The dermojet, which is recommended when large numbers of vaccinations have to be done, is a small pistol-like injector which squirts a stream of vaccine on to the skin at very high pressure.

After vaccination, excess lymph is wiped off with sterile cotton wool and the site allowed to dry. It is not necessary to apply a dressing at this stage. The patient should be advised to avoid wetting the site and a dry dressing should be applied if a pustule develops.

Three types of reaction may occur:

In the **primary reaction**, seen in persons not previously vaccinated, a red papule appears in 3–4 days. A vesicle develops in 5–6 days, becoming pustular in 8 days. After 11 days a dry scab has usually formed and this falls off after about 21 days.

The **accelerated reaction**, occurring only in persons previously vaccinated successfully, is similar but more rapid. The vesicle is formed on the third day and becomes pustular next day and the scab is off within 8 days.

An **immediate reaction** consists of an erythematous papule appearing usually within 24 hours and reaching a maximum in 72 hours, when it fades rapidly without the formation of a vesicle. This occurs only in persons previously vaccinated, and is a type IV hypersensitivity reaction. It does not necessarily indicate immunity although it often occurs in immune subjects.

A primary or accelerated reaction is associated with a sore arm during the vesicular and pustular stages. There is usually little or no general malaise, although small children may appear temporarily upset, but some restriction of activity is necessary and children should be forbidden vigorous games. The lesion is infectious at the pustular stage and patients should be advised accordingly.

Serious complications occasionally occur; the incidence of complications is least if primary vaccination is performed during the second year of life. Encephalitis and generalised vaccinia have already been mentioned. In persons with a history of dermatitis, the local reaction may be severe and constitute **eczema vaccinatum**. Necrosis of the skin may occur; this may be progressive in patients with hypogammaglobulinaemia or in patients receiving immunosuppressive drugs and is known as **vaccinia gangrenosa**.

Primary vaccination usually confers a good immunity for 5–10 years. Revaccination every 7 years has been the orthodox advice for a long time and this is sensible, but vaccination should have been carried out within 3 years if an assurance of protection is sought after there has been directed contact with a case of smallpox or during an epidemic. An international certificate of vaccination, which may be needed for travel between some countries, must be renewed every 3 years.

Influenza. Vaccines containing influenza viruses A and B inactivated with formaldehyde are available, but these are effective only against a limited range of antigenic variants of the virus. As immunisation provides little protection against the common small outbreaks of the disease that are due to numerous and often unidentified strains of virus, it is seldom used as a routine. In the event of a major epidemic due to a single strain of virus, a mass immunisation programme would be likely to give a large measure of protection to the community, provided that there was no unexpected antigenic change in the causative virus. A case can be made for giving the vaccine to those who are at special risk, for example elderly people in residential establishments, and also doctors and nurses.

Subunit flu vaccines have been developed in which the flu virus has been treated with detergent to release the superficial components of major antigenic significance. These 'split' vaccine preparations seems to be promising (see also p. 125).

Rabies vaccines. These are inactivated preparations of the virus harvested from (1) human or animal cells cultures, (2) duck embryo tissue, or (3) animal CNS tissue after laboratory infection with rabies. Adverse reactions to CNS tissue led to strenuous efforts to develop the less dangerous cell culture and duck embryo preparations. Courses of active immunisation given to a person after exposure to the risk of rabies range from 3–21 doses by subcutaneous injection. In cases of severe exposure, passive immunisation with rabies antiserum may also be advisable.

Plague and typhus (louse-borne). Vaccines are available for use in the event of an outbreak and are valuable for protection of members of the medical services.

Autogenous vaccines. At one time it was fashionable to treat patients suffering from chronic infections, especially of the skin and upper respiratory tract, with vaccines prepared from organisms isolated from the lesions. Clinical trials were seldom carried out and autogenous vaccines are now rarely made.

Developments
There is now promising research on new vaccines, e.g. for protection against cytomegalovirus infection, malaria, meningococcal meningitis, pseudomonas infection, bacillary dysentery, viral hepatitis and syphilis, but in 1982 none of these was in general use.

Passive immunisation
Passive immunity against some diseases can be conferred by injecting specific antibodies obtained from the serum of a convalescent patient or from a previously immunised animal. The extra circulating antibodies, added to those that might be naturally produced, may help to curtail an infection or neutralise a toxin and so moderate the illness. Passive immunisation has the disadvantages that it provides only temporary protection and, if an animal serum is used,

it is liable to provoke hypersensitivity reactions that range from a minor upset to severe anaphylaxis (p. 182).

In practice, passive immunisation has been most effectively exploited in the prophylaxis or treatment of infections caused by bacteria that produce exotoxins, such as diphtheria, botulism, tetanus and gas gangrene. Antisera against other bacteria have been prepared; effective antipneumococcal sera became available just before the introduction of sulphonamides, which proved to be much more effective, less hazardous and cheaper. Today, except for the antitoxic sera, the use of antisera is limited. Passive immunisation may be more useful in the future, especially for the prevention or treatment of conditions for which no effective antibiotic therapy is available. At present, antisera or gamma globulin preparations are available for the prevention or moderation of measles in debilitated children, rubella acquired in pregnancy, herpes zoster, vaccinia, viral hepatitis A and B, rabies, and anthrax. Antitoxic sera are also available for the therapy of some snake bites.

Reactions and contra-indications

In general, active immunisation with any vaccine should be postponed if the patients is temporarily unwell. If more than one live vaccine is to be given, there should be an interval of at least 3 weeks between them. Live vaccines should not be given to patients whose defences are compromised by malignant disease, severe chronic disease or immunodeficiency; this includes those receiving steroid therapy or cytotoxic therapy. Live viral vaccines, and especially rubella vaccine, should not be given during pregnancy.

Patients should be asked if they have previously reacted adversely to a vaccine and such a history should be taken into account before administering the vaccine again. This is of special importance in relation to pertussis vaccine and in cases of reactions to passive immunisation with heterologous antisera when there may be a danger of serious anaphylaxis.

Local erythema and tenderness at the injection site are common minor reactions. Fever, headache and malaise for a day or so occur in some people, especially after endotoxin-containing vaccines such as TAB or after a prolonged series of doses of cholera vaccine. Immune adults tend to react adversely to diphtheria immunisation. Children with a history or a family history of neonatal cerebral irritation, or a tendency to convulsions or epilepsy, or a previous reaction to pertussis vaccine should not receive the pertussis component of triple vaccine and should be given only the diphtheria-tetanus toxoids.

FURTHER READING

Ada G L 1981 Controlling influenza epidemics. Immunology Today 2: 219
Blackwell C C, Weir D M 1981 Principles of infection and immunity in patient care.
  Churchill Livingstone, Edinburgh
Bulletin of the World Health Organisation 1972 Virus-associated immunopathology:
  animal models and implications for human disease. Bulletin of WHO 47: 257
Bulletin of the World Health Organisation 1974 Immunology of schistosomiasis.
  Bulletin of WHO 51: 553
Collee J G 1981 Applied medical microbiology, 2nd edn. Blackwell, Oxford
Cox F E. G 1982 Cell-mediated immunity in theileriosis. Nature 295: 14
Dick G (ed) 1979 Immunological aspects of infectious disease. MTP Press, London
Evans D G 1969 Immunisation against infectious diseases. British Medical Bulletin
  25: 2
Fauci A S 1978 Host defence mechanisms against infection. Scope publication.
  Upjohn, Michigan
Gell P G H, Coombs R R A, Lachmann P J (eds) 1975 Clinical aspects of
  immunology, 3rd edn. Blackwell, Oxford
Hobson D 1967 Immunisation against respiratory virus infection. In: Cruickshank
  R, Weir D M (eds) Modern trends in immunology. Butterworth, London, vol 2,
  p 53
Notkins A L, Koprowski H 1973 How the immune response to a virus can cause
  disease. Scientific American 228: 22
Torrigiani G, Bell R (eds) 1981 Immunological recognition and effector mechanisms
  in infectious diseases. Schwabe, Basel
Voller A, Friedman H (eds) 1978 New trends and developments in vaccines. MTP
  Press, London
World Health Organisation 1975 Developments in malaria immunology. WHO
  Technical report series no. 579
Youmans G P, Paterson P Y, Somers H M (eds) 1975 The biological and clinical
  basis of infectious diseases. Saunders, Philadelphia

6

Immunohaematology

Objectives

On completion of this section the reader will be able to:

1. Draw up a table of the ABO blood group system indicating the antigens and isohaemagglutinins found in each of the groups A, B, O, and AB
2. Define 'universal donor'
3. Describe the phenomenon of Rhesus incompatibility and how the consequences can be abrogated
4. Describe the antiglobulin test
5. Outline the consequences of leucocyte incompatibility in transfusion
6. Give an example of a situation in which platelets may be given by transfusion

Knowledge of blood groups in man and animals has been very closely associated with the development of the science of immunology. Differences between the red blood cells of animals were first noted in goats as early as 1900 when Ehrlich and Morgenroth immunized 'a strong male goat' with nearly a litre of blood obtained from three other goats. The serum which they obtained from the immunized goat lysed the cells of all but one of the nine goats they tested. However, to Ehrlich the most important finding was that the cells of the immunized goat itself were completely unaffected. This proved to him that an animal would not produce autoantibodies against its own tissues and so destroy itself. It was left to Karl Landsteiner, who made the same observations in humans, to take up the detailed study of these antigenic differences. Landsteiner's important work on the immunological determinants of antigenic specificity stems from this period and still stands today as of fundamental value to our understanding of antigens.

Studies in blood group serology have led to the development of a large variety of techniques which have wide application to immunological problems outside this field. Notable amongst these is the antiglobulin test devised by Coombs and his associates, by means of which enormous advances have been made in many branches of immunology. Study of the development of blood group antibodies in serum has thrown light on the mechanisms underlying the formation of natural antibodies. Apart from these contributions to the understanding of immunological problems, information on blood groups has important implications in genetics and in forensic studies.

As has been noted in Chapter 5 (p. 117), blood group status appears to be associated with susceptibility to infections such as cholera (blood group O), gonorrhoea (blood group B) and *E. coli* infections of the urinary tract (groups B and AB). The reasons for these associations are not clear but may be related to cross-reactions between isohaemagglutinins or isoantibodies (see below) and cell wall antigens of various microorganisms. Such natural antibodies may act by blocking attachment of the bacterium to its target cell.

Blood groups

ABO antigens and isoantibodies

The ABO blood group system was described as a result of Landsteiner's demonstration of four distinct groups of agglutination reaction between human red blood cells and normal human serum. The differences in agglutination were due to the presence or absence of two antigens A and B on the red cell membrane. The four combinations which result from this are: (1) the presence of A antigen in the absence of B — group A cells; (2) the presence of B antigen in the absence of A — group B cells; (3) the presence of both A and B antigens — group AB cells; and (4) the absence of both A and B antigens — group O cells.

The sera of individuals also contain natural antibodies able to react with, and agglutinate if present in sufficient concentration, the cells of other individuals of different blood group.

These natural antibodies or **isoantibodies** are formed shortly after birth and appear to be stimulated by immunization with A and B antigens derived from the normal bacterial flora of the gut. Antigens with blood group specificity are widely distributed in nature (see also p. 28).

From a consideration of the phenomenon of immunological tolerance and the fact that an individual is tolerant to 'self' antigens (Ch. 9), it can be seen that an individual will respond only to an antigen to which he is not already tolerant. Thus an individual with blood group A cells will be tolerant to the A antigen and will therefore respond only to the B antigen derived from the gut flora. The

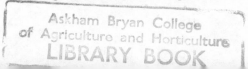

same holds for blood group B individuals who can respond only to the A antigen.

Thus individuals of blood group A will have isoantibodies of blood group B specificity, i.e. anti-B antibodies, and blood group B individuals will in the same way have anti-A isoantibodies. Blood group O individuals whose immune system will not have developed tolerance to either A or B antigens will have, as would be expected, both anti-A and anti-B isoagglutinins.

The blood group antigens A and B occur not only in the red cells but are widely distributed in the tissues with the exception of the central nervous system. Just under 80% of individuals also have one of these antigens (corresponding to their blood group) in the tissue fluids and secretions (except CSF). Chemical studies on these antigens recovered in quantity from ovarian cyst fluid show them to be glycoproteins and that the difference between A and B substances is determined by the nature of a single saccharide attached to the terminal sugar of the glycoprotein chain. Group O individuals secrete a glycoprotein (H-substance) which is probably the basic chain structure material from which A and B substances are derived by the addition of the specific saccharides (p. 30).

Blood transfusion in relation to ABO groups

Transfusion of an individual with red cells from an individual of a different group results in exposure of the transfused cells to an isoagglutinin — anti-A or anti-B — and except in the case of O cells which carry neither the A nor the B antigen, the cells will be destroyed with resulting haemoglobinaemia and haemoglobinuria. Although it is clearly best to administer blood only of the same group as the recipient, in an emergency group O cells can be given. Although the plasma of a group O individual (sometimes called a 'universal donor') contains anti-A and anti-B isoagglutinins, these are so diluted by the recipient's plasma (a pint of blood would be diluted about 1 in 12) to have only a negligible effect except when large quantities of blood have to be administered. Group O individuals whose serum contains anti-A and anti-B isoagglutinins cannot accept blood of any group except O. Since an individual of group AB has neither anti-A nor anti-B isoantibodies he can accept blood of any of the four groups and has therefore been called a 'universal recipient'.

This relatively straightforward scheme is unfortunately slightly complicated by the existence of a number of subgroups of A (probably five in all). However, only A_1 and A_2 are of importance as far as transfusion is concerned. The frequency of occurrence in Caucasians of the six different ABO groups is shown below.

Blood group	Frequency	Isoantibodies
O	43.5%	Anti-A (+ Anti-A$_1$), Anti-B
A$_1$	34.8%	Anti-B
A$_2$	9.6%	Anti-B (occasionally Anti-A$_1$)
B	8.5%	Anti-A (+ Anti-A$_1$)
A$_1$B	2.5%	None
A$_2$B	0.8%	None (occasionally Anti-A$_1$)

The Rhesus blood group system

This system is the next most important system to the ABO groups. The Rh blood group antigens are present in the red cells of 85% of Caucasians and 94% of Negroes. The most common of the Rhesus antigens are C, c, D, d, E, e, and the table below shows some of the various combinations which can exist and their frequency in Caucasians.

Genotype	Frequency	
CDe/cde	31.7%	
CDe/CDe	16.6%	
CDe/cDe	11.5%	Rh-positive
cDE/cde	10.9%	
cde/cde	15.1%	Rh-negative

The Rhesus group of an individual must be taken into account for transfusion purposes. Of these antigens D is the most potent although immunization by D and at the same time by the C or E antigens can occur. A variant of D named D^u has been described and cells carrying this antigen are not agglutinated by routine anti-D sera. For transfusion purposes recipients carrying the D^u antigen are considered to be Rh-negative, whilst donors in this category are regarded as Rh-positive.

Rhesus incompatibility

The clinical importance of the Rhesus groups lies in the ability of the red cells of a Rhesus-positive fetus to immunize its Rhesus-negative mother. Immunization usually takes place following the trauma of parturition with the result that the maternal immune response does not develop until a **second** pregnancy. The maternal anti-Rh antibody is passed to the new fetus via the placenta and causes haemolytic destruction of its erythrocytes. This condition is known as **haemolytic disease of the newborn** or erythroblastosis fetalis. Since the original description of the disease it has been found that blood group antigen systems other than the Rh system can be responsible for the condition. For example a group O mother can occasionally be immunized by fetal antigens if the father is A_1, A_1B or B.

The serious nature of haemolytic disease of the newborn necessitating complete exchange of the infant's blood (exchange transfusion) to remove the maternal antibody, has now been alleviated by a rather ingenious immunological manoeuvre. This is based on the observation that attempted immunization by an antigen in the presence of its specific antibody tends to inhibit synthesis of the antibody to the injected antigen. It is known, for example, that immunization of infants is best delayed for a few months after birth to allow the levels of maternal antibody to fall.

In the case of a recognized Rhesus incompatibility it is now the practice to give a small dose of potent anti-Rh antibody to immunized Rh-negative mothers within three days after delivery of an Rh-positive infant. The antibody appears to inhibit the response to the Rhesus antigen, possibly by diverting the cells carrying the antigen from the antibody-forming tissues or perhaps by a direct 'feedback inhibition' effect on the antibody-forming cells. This treatment has been very successful in clinical trials and the future outlook is very hopeful so that the disease may soon become of only historical interest (Fig. 6.1).

The detection of anti-Rh antibodies

After the recognition of the association between haemolytic disease of the newborn and Rhesus immunization, it soon became apparent that the standard method of demonstrating anti-Rh antibody — by direct agglutination of a saline suspension of Rh-positive cells by serum from an immunized mother — was not able to show up the presence of antibody in one-half to two-thirds of sera tested. A solution to the problem was found by the substitution of a dilute protein solution, e.g. bovine albumen, for the normal saline diluent. Visible agglutination could then be readily demonstrated in the majority of cases. The form of serum antibody responsible for agglutination, demonstrable only in protein diluent, became known

1.

FATHER
Rhesus +ve

MOTHER
Rhesus -ve

Rhesus
antigen
immunizes
mother

1st. Child
Normal

INFANT
Rhesus +ve

Maternal
anti-Rhesus
antibody

2nd. Child
Haemolytic anaemia
anaemia

INFANT
Rhesus +ve

Maternal
anti-Rhesus
antibody

2.

FATHER
Rhesus +ve

MOTHER
Rhesus -ve

Anti-Rhesus serum
to mother blocks
immunization

1st. Child
Normal

INFANT
Rhesus +ve

Rhesus
antigen

2nd. Child
Normal

INFANT
Rhesus +ve

Fig. 6.1 Scheme showing consequence of immunization of Rhesus −ve mother by
Rhesus antigen of Rhesus +ve child. Prevention obtained by injection of
anti-Rhesus serum after delivery of first child

as 'incomplete' antibody in contrast to the saline-active 'complete'
antibody. The incomplete antibody was thought of initially as uni-
valent, having only one antibody-binding site, but it has now been
shown to be IgG antibody of normal bivalent structure (p. 65); the
complete anti-red cell antibody, on the other hand, has been shown
to be IgM in nature. It seems that the smaller molecular weight IgG
antibody is not readily able to link together red cells in suspension
unless the mutually repellent effect of red cells, which normally
keeps them in suspension in a saline medium, is reduced by altering their surface charge by the addition of protein. In contrast the
much larger, multivalent IgM antibodies have a considerably
greater chance of bringing about agglutination.

Another very important method for demonstrating incomplete
antibodies is the Coombs **antiglobulin test**. An antiserum is prepared in rabbits against human immunoglobulins and this is used to
react with Rh-positive cells, coated with human incomplete antibody, bringing about their agglutination simply by linking together

the molecules of human globulin still attached to the red cells (p. 230 and Fig. 10.9).

One of the advantages of this method is that it can be used to detect the coating in vivo of Rh-positive cells by small amounts of antibody. After the cells have been thoroughly washed, they are mixed with the anti-human globulin serum which will bring about agglutination of cells with human globulin attached to their surface. This form of the test is known as the 'direct Coombs test'. Another form of the test is used to detect incomplete anti-Rh antibodies in the serum of a patient who has been immunized against Rh antigens. Rh-positive cells are simply mixed with the patient's serum and if anti-Rh antibody is present the cells will be agglutinated by the subsequent addition of an anti-human globulin serum. This variation is known as the 'indirect Coombs test'.

Maternal responses to other fetal antigens

In addition to responding to the Rhesus antigen the mother can respond to other blood group antigens, and mothers lacking the A or B red cell antigen who carry a fetus possessing such antigen will probably develop raised levels of anti-A or anti-B isoagglutinins. Such sera are useful for blood typing purposes, as are sera containing anti-HLA antibodies which are often found in multiparous women and which can be used for leucocyte typing. Spermatozoa, although they carry histocompatibility antigens, rarely seem to immunize. Immunization of the mother to fetal antigen probably occurs following passage of fetal blood (by small haemorrhages) into the maternal bloodstream and occurs more frequently as pregnancy progresses. The fetus represents an allograft containing potentially immunogenic antigens derived from paternal antigens of the major histocompatibility complex (MHC). The mother makes both humoral and cell-mediated responses to these antigens but the fetus survives because the placenta appears to be an immunologically privileged site and does not allow effector cells or antibodies to affect fetal development. The placenta seems to be able to absorb out antifetal antibodies from the maternal blood and H-2K and H-2D antigens of paternal type have been found on the mouse placenta. There is evidence that MHC disaparity is associated with fetal survival. Women who have chronic abortions share more HLA antigens with their husbands than predicted by chance. The placenta is believed to be responsible for balancing the tendency for rejection of the fetus with 'facilitation' that allows the fetus to survive to term. In man (but not mouse) the trophoblast lacks MHC antigens.

A number of pregnancy-associated substances a such as alpha-fetoprotein 17β-oestradiol, prostaglandin synthetase inhibitor and β_1-microglobulin may play a role in regulating the immune response in pregnancy. It has also been found that natural killer cells (p. 130) are absent in neonates. It is becoming apparent that a certain degree of foreignness may actually assist human reproduction and viviparity. An IgG 'blocking factor' has been found in maternal serum that inhibits production of lymphokines by maternal lymphocytes sensitized to antigens on the trophoblast and paternal lymphocytes. Women who undergo recurrent abortions of unknown aetiology lack the blocking factor. Preliminary trials in which 'blocking factor' is induced by immunization with pooled leucocyte infusions have resulted in encouraging results.

Other blood group systems
In 1927 Landsteiner described two human antigens, M and N. The use of antisera against these antigens can divide individuals into three types, half having the MN genotype and 28% and 22% respectively having MM and NN genotypes. A further antigen was later found, the S antigen, and the group is known as the MNS blood group system. This group is of limited clinical importance although a few instances of haemolytic disease of the newborn have been reported due to incompatibility of these antigens.

Landsteiner's P antigen is noteworthy because a naturally occurring anti-P cold agglutinin is found in a large proportion of the 20% of individuals who are P-negative. Amongst a number of blood group systems described including those of Lutheran, Kell, Lewis, Kidd, Duffy and Diego, special mention should be made of the Lewis system because naturally occurring antibodies to Lewis antigens are frequently found in human serum. They sometimes act as cold agglutinins and have been found occasionally to be the cause of haemolytic transfusion reactions. These antigens are unique in that they are not part of the red cell structure but are soluble antigens found in body fluids, which adsorb on to the red cell surface.

Antigens of blood leucocytes and platelets
As will be discussed in the section on transplantation antigens, blood leucocytes in man carry the major histocompatibility antigen system HLA. The appearance of antibodies against donor leucocytes and also platelet antigens is a common finding after blood transfusion. This results in rapid destruction of the transfused cells and although immunization occurs more frequently than anti-red cell immunization the consequences are less dangerous.

Leucocyte and platelet groups fall into two types: those which they share in common with red cells, and those with antigens which are restricted to leucocytes and platelets and other tissue cells. The blood group antigens A and B are the main antigens shared with erythrocytes. The important antigenic group is limited to leucocytes, platelets and other tissue cells in the HLA system.

A reaction between anti-leucocyte isoantibodies and transfused leucocytes often gives rise to febrile transfusion reactions and their incidence can be correlated with the number of transfusions given. Although these reactions are not usually severe they can be a disadvantage to patients for whom repeated transfusions are necessary. In this situation the simplest solution is to remove the majority of leucocytes from the blood by separation of red cells which can be readily sedimented by the addition of gelatin. This is preferable to the complex serological procedures required to assure compatibility of leucocytes.

The transfusion of fresh platelets is of value in patients suffering from haemorrhagic disorders due to thrombocytopenia, and although theoretically, selection of compatible platelets is desirable, in practice platelets are usually obtained from a small number of donors, if possible related to the recipient.

The HLA system of antigens is of considerable current interest to immunologists because of their importance as histocompatibility antigens. Unfortunately the HLA system appears to be a most complex system but with wide implications in immunology. It is the equivalent of the H-2 system in the mouse and of the other main histocompatibility systems known to exist in other mammalian species (see p. 98).

Between 15 and 20 more or less well-defined antigens have been identified in the HLA system, and more than 100 phenotypes have been found within this system. Despite these complexities, as more experience is gained in the grouping procedures (leucoagglutination by a panel of antisera) and supplies of suitable antisera become more widely available, it seems likely that by accumulating a list of available fully typed donors and with improvements in storage and preservation of tissues, it may eventually become possible to select from amongst the many possible variations a suitable donor for each recipient.

FURTHER READING

Bulletin of the World Health Organization 1967 The suppression of Rh-immunization by passively administered human immunoglobulin (IgG) anti-D (anti-Rh$_0$). Bulletin of WHO 36: 467

Dausset J, Colombani J 1967 White cells and platelets in transfusion immunology. In: Cruickshank R, Weir D M (eds) Modern trends in immunology. Butterworth, London, vol 2, p 314

Dodd B E, Lincoln P J 1975 Blood group topics. In: Turk J L (ed) Current topics in immunology. Arnold, London, vol 3

Race R R, Sanger R 1975 Blood groups in man, 6th edn. Blackwell, Oxford

Singh B, Gambel P 1982, Reproduction: protection and prevention! Immunology Today 3:1

Stern C M 1975 Feto-maternal relationships. In: Hobart M J, McConnell I (eds) The Immune system, Blackwell, Oxford

7

The immunology of tissue transplantation

Objectives
On completion of this section the reader will be able to:
1. Describe, in outline form, the transplantation antigen systems of man and the mouse and how these antigens are detected
2. Define 'first set' and 'second set' graft rejection
3. Outline the role of lymphocytes and humoral antibody in graft rejection
4. Describe two approaches to immunosuppression.

The tissue cells of animals contain antigens that are specific for the species of origin of the cell, and which if implanted into an animal of another species will induce an immune response. This response rapidly destroys the implanted cells and has the characteristics of the primary and secondary immune response as already described for antigens in general. In addition to species-specific antigens, differences also exist between individual members of the same species so that transfer of tissue cells between members induces a similar immune reaction. The closer the relationship between two individuals of the same species, the more likely are implanted cells to survive. In the case of identical twins survival is assured. Inbred strains of animals, particularly mice, have been de-

Table 7.1 Transplantation terminology (older terminology in brackets)

Relationship between donor and recipient	Term applied to relationship	Prefix applied to graft, antigen or antibody
Of different species	Xenogeneic (heterogeneic)	Xeno- (hetero-)
Of same species but different genetic constitution	Allogeneic (homologous)	Allo- (homo-)
Of same inbred strain	Syngeneic (isogeneic) (isologous)	–
Same individual	Autologous	Auto-

veloped which are genetically identical and these are widely used in experimental work on tissue transplantation immunology.

In man surgical techniques are available to enable transplantation of many organs and tissues but unfortunately a high proportion of organ transplants fail because of rejection by the immune response or because of the side effects of attempts to suppress the immune response, due to toxicity of the drugs or their depressive effect on resistance to infection.

Transplantation antigen systems

The first systematic studies on the antigens carried by cells which determine whether a graft will be rejected or not were carried out in inbred strains of mice of known genetic make-up.

It was found that there were very many antigenic differences between tissues of different strains of mice, the number of separate antigens involved being estimated at between 15 and 500 in different experiments. However, it was found that, just as in the red cell antigenic system, some antigens were very 'strong' and others very weak. The strong transplantation or 'histocompatibility' antigens of the mouse are controlled by the H-2 genetic locus and in man by the HLA locus.

The mouse H-2 system appears to consist of a system of closely linked genes and there are hundreds of possible combinations resulting in different H-2 antigens. H-2 antigens are found in large amounts in epithelium and lymphoid tissues, in very small amounts in kidney or muscle and are virtually absent from brain and testis.

In man, two strong and several weak histocompatibility systems have been found. As mentioned already, the HLA is the strong system with the ABH blood group system next in importance. The major loci are very complex, the antigens being determined by a chromosomal region rather than by a single gentic locus.

Chemical studies on soluble H-2 antigens have shown them to be glycoproteins. Analysis of the amino acid constitution of extracted transplantation antigen of two different inbred strains of guinea-pig indicates that they are distinct.

HLA-A and HLA-B of chromosome 6 (Fig. 7.1a) are the human counterpart of the mouse H-2K and H-2D loci and are the antigens most often used in immune typing. This is done with a panel of various monospecific HLA antisera, often obtained from women who had multiple pregnancies or, increasingly, with monoclonal antibodies prepared against HLA antigens.

The test is carried out with lymphocytes from the individual to be typed incubated with the various antisera and complement. The presence of a particular antigen on the surface of the lymphocyte, in the presence of appropriate antibody and complement, leads to lysis of the lymphocyte. Lysis is detected by the failure of the cell to exclude the dye trypan blue (see p. 234).

Different HLA-A and HLA-B antigens are given numbers, e.g. HLA-B5. No individual has more than 2 HLA-A antigen specifications and 2 HLA-B antigen specifications. Thus an individual heterogenous at each locus can express four major HLA specificities, two from each parent.

A further locus, the HLA-D locus, appears to be the equivalent of the I region in the mouse. As in the mouse it is involved in various lymphocyte activating functions. The HLA-C locus is of lesser importance than HLA-A and HLA-B in graft rejection as it determines relatively weak transplantation antigens.

Grafts between HLA identical siblings are the most successful and have a greater chance of survival than HLA-A and HLA-B matched grafts that are not neccessarily identical at other loci.

Figure 7.1b shows the structure of the human HLA antigens indicating the two-chain arrangement including β_2 microglobulin. The larger component of 44 000 daltons molecular weight contains amino acid sequences that show some homology with the constant domains of the immunoglobulin G molecule.

Fig. 7.1a Human major histocompatibility region

Fig. 7.1b Human HLA transmembrane glycoprotein, showing structure of A, B and C antigens. β_2 microglobulin is not coded for by MHC region

Leucocyte grouping. The strong antigens of the HLA system are widely distributed in the tissues but absent from the red blood cells which contain only the ABH antigens.

Fortunately blood leucocytes carry all the known HLA antigens and it is therefore possible to test for the presence or absence of antigens of the system using leucocyte agglutination and cyto-toxicity tests (p. 234). In principle the leuco-agglutination test is performed with leucocytes separated from the erythrocytes of anti-coagulant-treated blood. Specific antisera for HLA antigens are then used to agglutinate the leucocytes and the tests are read under the microscope. The cytotoxic test is carried out with a purified suspension of blood lymphocytes which are mixed with antisera to HLA antigens in the presence of complement (p. 235). If the lymphocytes carry the appropriate antigens the antiserum will combine and in the presence of complement will damage the cell membrane. The resulting increased cell membrane permeability is usually detected by dye uptake into the cell. Matching donor and recipient for HLA antigens, including the DR antigens (the human equivalent of the mouse Ia antigens), is normally carried out prior to grafting.

Despite the very great diversity among HLA alleles of unrelated subjects it is encouraging to find that about a third of kidneys from unrelated donors survive for a year or longer although only a third of them show normal kidney function. Although this partial success must be dependent to an extent on the use of immunosuppressive agents, differences in the 'strength' of individual HLA antigens is probably partly responsible.

Mechanisms of graft rejection

There are two main types of graft rejection process: (a) the so-called 'first set' response which occurs about 10 days after a first graft from an unrelated donor, (b) the 'second set' response occurring in about 7 days in an animal which had previously received a graft from the same unrelated donor. This phenomenon of first and second set rejection can be compared to primary and secondary immunization — the accelerated secondary response being brought about by stimulation of an already sensitized or 'primed' immune system.

The role of lymphoid cells. It can be shown histologically that grafts undergoing rejection are heavily infiltrated with lymphocytes and that there is extensive vascular damage. Other types of cells of the immune system, such as plasma cells and macrophages, are also frequently found in association with graft rejection. The ability to

Fig. 7.2 Schematic view of rejection mechanisms and their prevention

reject grafts can readily be transferred from one animal to another by a process known as **adoptive transfer** of lymphoid cells from an immune animal (i.e. one capable of a second set graft rejection) to a non-immune recipient of the same strain. Lymphoid cells appear to be able to transfer this ability most effectively when taken before the circulating antibody level reaches its peak. Contrary to expectation, it is possible to show, using isotope-labelled cells, that it is not the transferred cells which migrate to the graft but those of the recipient. The donated cells in the main home to the lymphoid organs, as no more are found in the graft than at control sites. It is, however, possible that those few donated cells which settle in the graft area are cells specifically sensitised to the graft antigens whilst those settling out elsewhere are the unsensitised cells.

From what is known about the recirculating lymphocyte pool (p. 96), it seems likely that there is a good chance of cells with a specific ability to react to an antigen coming in contact with such material in a graft during the process of lymphocyte recirculation. Donor lymphocytes carried over as 'passengers' in the vascular bed of the graft could be a source of transplantation antigens that could sensitize the host. In rats pretreatment of donors with immunosuppressive agents to deplete the lymphocyte population resulted in prolongation of graft survival. Stimulation of the host cells residing in the lymphoid organs would be excepted if they came in contact with transplantation antigens carried by passenger lymphocytes from the graft, as described above, which themselves reach the spleen.

The role of circulating antibody. The ability to reject grafts cannot be transferred from one animal to another by means of passively injected antibody. This does not rule out the possibility that antibody can play a part in graft rejection, because when the serum, containing at best about 1% specific antibody, is injected into a recipient the diluting effect of the blood and tissue fluids considerably reduces the possibility of the antibody reaching the graft site in an adequate concentration to influence the viability of the graft. The same antibody-containing serum can readily be shown in vitro to be cytotoxic, in the presence of complement, for cells containing antigens to which the antibody was produced. However, this is an artificial situation and does not take into account the dilution effects discussed above. Kidney grafts which have survived for some time, perhaps months or years, can, it seems, be rejected by serum antibody alone without any evidence of invasion of the graft by lymphoid cells. Deposits of immunoglobulin and complement can be detected particularly in the walls of blood vessels. Although at this stage no antibodies may be detected in the serum, if the rejected kidney is removed they soon appear, suggesting that the antibodies were rapidly removed by combination with kidney antigens. The kidney is rejected by the development of a progressive vasculitis affecting glomerular and other vessels. Attempts have been made to recover antibody by elution from rejected kidneys removed from 27 patients. Seven of the kidneys contained recoverable antibody and this often differed from that found in the patient's serum, supporting the view that grafted incompatible kidneys filter out antibody from the circulation.

Locally produced antibody and non-antibody lymphocyte factors. The possibility is quite strong that antibody made locally in a graft by the infiltrating lymphoid cells is present in a sufficiently high concentration in the area immediately surrounding the antibody-producing cell to damage incompatible cells of the graft. This situation can be compared to the observation made in vitro with the Jerne plaque technique (p. 58) in which lymphocytes can be shown to be producing antibody to sheep red blood cells which produces a surrounding halo of lysis of the red cells in the presence of complement. Indeed, lymphocytes and plasma cells invading grafts can be shown to contain immunoglobulin. Evidence that immunoglobulin is combining with antigen during graft rejection is provided by a detectable fall in the serum complement level.

There are a number of other possible direct ways in which the infiltrating lymphocytes can influence survival of the graft: (a) the antibody which they produce may activate the various pharmacological mediators of immediate hypersensitivity reactions such as histamine (p. 183) and these will bring about changes in the vessels of the graft: (b) the lymphocytes on contact with antigen may release macrophage migration inhibition factor (MIF) (p. 93) which will cause accumulation of macrophages in the graft; (c) it is known that sensitised lymphocytes can influence non-immune lymphocytes to behave aggressively towards cells in their vicinity and induce cytoxic effects.

Experimental evidence has shown that only a low percentage of the lymphocytes infiltrating a graft are specifically reactive to graft alloantigens. Lymphokines secreted by helper T lymphocytes may be responsible for the migration and proliferation of the majority of the infiltrating inflammatory cells. Graft rejection can be inhibited by in vivo administration of antisera against lymphokines. Adoptive transfer experiments in T lymphocyte-depleted mice indicate that Ly-1 helper T cells are critical to skin-graft rejection in mice. Furthermore, injections of interleukin 2 (a helper T cell product) can greatly enhance heart graft rejection in rats.

Other cell types may influence graft rejection and it has been found that monocytes and macrophages accumulate in large numbers early in human renal graft rejection.

It can thus be seen that the reaction against a graft depends upon a complex series of interrelated phenomena, some of which are specifically induced by the foreign nature of graft antigens. Other phenomena are non-specific in the immunological sense and occur as part of an inflammatory process.

Immunosuppression

Graft rejection, as has been noted, involves a sequence of separate phenomena developing from initial contact of the foreign antigens with the host immunological system through to rejection itself. The steps include establishment of lymphatic drainage, antigen release, its contact with cells of the immune system, proliferation of antibody-forming cells of the lymphoid tissues, the inflammatory response and release of pharmacological mediators and cytotoxic effects of lymphoid cells and/or antibody on the graft tissues.

Prevention of sensitization; tolerance to graft antigens. Interference with any of these stages would be likely to interfere with the rejection process. One of the most interesting approaches, which is as yet unfortunately only at the experimental stage, is interference with what might be termed the afferent arc of the process of rejection, namely the initial sensitization of the lymphoid cells. If it were possible to induce immune tolerance (p. 87) to the strong histocompatibility antigens of tissue grafts, then immunological rejection would not take place. The tolerant animal, although unable to react against the antigen to which it is tolerant, can still respond to other antigens such as potentially infective agents like bacteria, fungi or viruses; this obviates one of the greatest difficulties associated with immunosuppressive procedures.

As has been noted earlier, Mitchison (using serum protein antigens) has shown that there are two types of tolerance, so-called 'high dose' tolerance where the immune system is overloaded with excess antigen, and 'low dose' tolerance where only minute quantities of antigen are administered. Although the molecular processes underlying these phenomena are not as yet understood, the 'low dose' tolerance phenomena has great potential application to transplantation problems. When it becomes possible to extract purified transplantation antigens from tissue, it should then be possible to prepare an individual for graft acceptance by inducing low dose tolerance to the appropriate antigens.

Some progress has been made recently in the induction of specific tolerance against transplantation antigens in rats by eliminating the T lymphocytes which normally respond to graft antigens. It has been done by preparing antibodies against the T cell receptors for the major histocompatibility antigens. This is achieved by mating two inbred strains of rat; the hybrids would express the histocompatibility antigens of each parent and thus be tolerant to them. The implication is that the T cells would not express receptors for the antigens whilst each of the parents would express receptors for the histocompatibility antigens of the other strain. Thus by injecting the hybrid rats with lymphocytes from a parent the hybrids would not react to the histocompatibility antigen but would react to the receptors for the antigen on the parental cells.

T lymphocytes shed their receptors and it is therefore possible to extract these for the major histocompatibility antigen by binding them to the antibody (attached to an inert particle). The purified T cell receptors are then chemically modified by cross linking with gluteraldehyde (to make them immunogenic). When these are injected into an inbred strain of rats (Lewis) with adjuvant, they are able to slow down the rejection of grafts from another inbred strain (DA). The eventual rejection of the graft in 24 days (compared to 11 days in untreated rats) is probably due to minor histocompatibility differences. The prolongation of graft survival is likely to be due to suppression or elimination of lymphocytes bearing the receptor for the major histocompatibility antigen by the antibodies induced by the chemically modified purified receptor.

Another approach at inducing transplantation tolerance is the repeated injection of massive doses of serum into neonatal rats. The serum contains small amounts of histocompatibility antigen and this is sufficient in neonatal rats to induce a lasting tolerance to certain skin grafts showing strong histocompatibility differences between donor and recipient. The practical value of this approach is clearly limited by the requirement that tolerance he induced in neonatal animals.

Immunological enhancement. Another phenomenon relevant to the maintenance of incompatible grafts is 'immunological enhancement'. This is brought about by antibody produced against graft antigens that can under certain circumstances protect the graft from attack by cells of the immune system. This system has been used successfully in rats with incompatible kidney grafts, the animals being previously immunized with tissue from the prospective donor. The grafts exhibit normal renal function for a year or more afterwards. The method has been applied in a few instances to human kidney grafts and the results suggest that the method may be of considerable future value. The mechanism may involve coating of the cells of the graft by non-complement-fixing antibody and/or direct inhibition of antibody production against the graft brought about by the antibody. The danger of the antibody damaging the graft will require the use of antisera (directed against the histocompatibility antigens) that has been treated so as to eliminate any cytotoxic effects. This could be achieved by making use of antibody fragments (Fab) that do not bind complement (p. 65).

Practical approaches. In practice there are at the moment three main approaches to the problem of immunosuppression: (1) X-irradiation to knock out the lymphoid tissues and abolish the immune response; (2) immuno-suppressive drugs — antimetabolites and anti-inflammatory agents to prevent proliferation of antibody-forming cells; (3) immunological methods — anti-lymphocyte serum (ALS) produced, for example, in the horse, to attack the lymphocytes directly and destroy them before they attack the graft.

Whole body X-irradiation used in the early days of organ transplantation has been replaced in the main by immunosuppressive drugs and ALS. Some attention has been given to reducing the lymphocyte count in the peripheral blood by passing it through an extracorporeal shunt and irradiating it outside the body. This method, although tried so far only on a small scale and with a limited degree of success, may be of value in the future. The drugs prednisone and Imuran (azathioprine) in combination are widely used and for immunosuppression are often given together with ALS. These substances in high dosage are toxic but haemodialysis before operation and during rejection crises reduces their toxicity in renal transplant cases. Cyclosporin A, a cyclic undecapeptide from *Trichoderma polysporum*, has been recently introduced and appears to be more specific in the target cells affected. It may however not be without toxic effects.

Any of these regimes clearly carries with it the considerable risk of infection and the commonest cause of death after kidney grafting is not graft rejection but infection with fungi, viruses and bacteria. Another apparent complication noted in the last few years is the small but significant increase in reticulosarcomata following prolonged immunosuppressive therapy. This could conceivably be due to inhibition of the immunological surveillance mechanism (Ch. 8).

Anti-lymphocyte serum has the advantage of primarily affecting the thymus-dependent lymphocytes of the spleen and lymph nodes, and lymphocytes circulating in the blood. This results in a suppression of the cell-mediated immune response with only a slight effect on the circulating antibody response. Thus, whilst suppressing the graft rejection mechanisms ALS leaves the animal able to produce circulating antibody against infecting microorganisms and their products. However, infections caused by intracellular agents such as viruses in which protection depends on cell-mediated immunity (p. 127) still remain a possible complication in this form of immunosuppression and different preparations of ALS may vary in their effect on the antibody response. Furthermore, ALS can destroy platelets because of shared platelet and leucocyte antigen and may require prior absorption with platelet suspensions. Anaphylactic reactions may occur because of the foreign nature of the protein and severe pain frequently occurs at the injection site.

Trials with monoclonal antibodies to lymphocyte antigens are underway in patients undergoing renal graft rejection. If these continue to prove successful then more specific monoclonal reagents directed at specific T cell subpopulations may prove to be more useful.

FURTHER READING

Bagshawe K D 1972 Immunosuppression. British Journal of Hospital Medicine 8: 677

Baldwin W H 1981 Do cytotoxic T lymphocytes cause transplant rejection? Immunology Today 2: 210

Berenabum M C 1967 Transplantation and immunosuppression. In: Cruickshank R, Weir D M (eds) Modern trends in immunology. Butterworth, London, vol 2, p 292

Carpenter C B 1981 Immunology Today 2: 50

James K 1967 Anti-lymphocyte antibody: a review. Clinical and Experimental
    Immunology 2: 615
Merrill J P 1967 Human tissue transplantation. Advances in Immunology 2: 615
Perkins H A 1976 Transplantation immunology. In: Fudenberg H H, Stites D P,
    Caldwell J L, Wells J V (eds) Basic and clinical immunology. Lange, Los Altos
Porter K A 1967 Symposium on tissue and organ transplantation. Journal of Clinical
    Pathology (supplement) 20: 415
Rapaport F T, Dausset J 1968 Human transplantation. Grune and Stratton, New
    York

8

Malignant disease

OBJECTIVES

On completion of this section the reader will be able to:

1. Give two examples implicating dificiency of the immune mechanisms in the development of tumours
2. define 'immune surveillance'
3. Give two examples of the two types of antigenic change found in tumours
4. Give two examples of agents used in tumour immunotherapy, their mode of action and their possible value.

In discussing the general biological significance of immune reactions in maintaining the integrity of the cellular systems of the body, Burnet points out that in man, in whom more than 10^{14} cells are constantly reproducing, there is sufficient evidence to make it likely that at any given genetic locus an error occurs with a frequency in the range of 10^{-5} to 10^{-7} per replication. This means that in the cell population there must be many millions of errors or mutations occurring every day of life. It seems inconceivable that complex and long-lived multicellular animals could have evolved unless some means of dealing with this eventuality had been developed. Recently, however, doubt has been expressed on this view and it has been suggested that 'this daily development of malignant cells is not supported by the experimental evidence, and that spontaneous malignant transformation in vitro appears to be dependent more on cell-to-cell interactions than to be an intrinsic property of single cells.'

The role of immunological mechanisms in the suppression of malignant cells has been appreciated since the work of Paul Ehrlich at the beginning of the century, but it is only in the last 10 years or so that immunologists have begun to unravel the details of the immunological processes underlying the control of tumours, the antigenic changes in tumour cells themselves, and the extent and activities of the immune response arising as a result of these changes.

Evidence for the role of immune mechanisms

Mention is made in Chapter 5 of the increased incidence in thymectomized mice of tumours induced by chemical carcinogens and viruses. This seems likely to be due to a deficiency of the cell-mediated immune mechanisms which are the control of the thymus (p. 44). These neonatally **thymectomized** animals are unable to reject incompatible tissue grafts and do not give delayed hypersensitivity reactions of the tuberculin type. These activities depend on intact cell-mediated, thymus-dependent immune reactivity and it is the absence of this reactivity which allows tumour cells to grow unhindered.

The experimental evidence in support of this view is conflicting. Thymectomy of mice does appear to increase the incidence of skin tumours to certain chemical carcinogens (polycyclic hydrocarbons) and of tumours induced by DNA viruses. However, early thymectomy seems to have no significant effect on development of spontaneous tumours in mice and there are reports of a decreased incidence of tumours, such as mouse mammary carcinoma, following thymectomy. It thus appears that the effects of thymectomy are variable and depend to some extent on other factors, such as the agent responsible for tumour development.

Another example where deficiency of the cell-mediated immune mechanisms is associated with tumour formation is in a condition known as **graft-versus-host** disease. This condition is produced in mice by injecting spleen cells into an unrelated recipient, the reaction of the spleen cells against the host resulting in destruction of its lymphoid tissues. This can be demonstrated by using two inbred strains of mice, e.g. CBA and C57 Black, and injecting the spleen cells of one of the parents into the offspring of such a mating. CBA cells injected into a CBA/C57B recipient will recognize the C57B component of the host-lymphoid cells as foreign but will not be themselves rejected because the recipient itself carries the CBA antigens.

The destruction of the recipient's lymphoid tissues, and thus its cell-mediated immune response, produces a defect in the control of neoplastic cell proliferation. These mice frequently develop tumours of the lymphoid tissues having many of the features of Hodgkin's disease of the human.

A herpes virus (Epstein-Barr) has been isolated from the human lymphoid tumour known as **Burkitt's lymphoma** and it has been proposed that the tumour is of virus origin. Recent evidence in patients with Burkitt's lymphoma has added considerable support to the significance of cell-mediated immunes mechanisms in the control of the tumour. Only one of 12 patients on skin testing with extracts of their own tumour cells had positive delayed hypersensitivity reactions. However, when the tumour growth was suppressed with cyclophosphamide, skin tests became positive in seven of the twelve indicating a recovery of the cell-mediated immune mechanisms which is associated with remission of the tumour.

Serological studies have demonstrated a strong association between the presence of high titres of antibody to EB virus in both Burkitt's lymphoma and postnasal carcinoma. However, antibody to the virus is widespread throughout the world and association can be found with a number of diverse disease states. The virus can be found not only in leucocytes of patients with Burkitt's lymphoma but also in leucocytes of patients with infectious mononucleosis and even in some normal individuals. The virus appears to be able in vitro to **transform** leucocytes into virus-containing cells capable of continuous growth. The virus appears to have a predilection for cells of the lymphoid organs and it cannot yet be excluded that the virus is a 'passenger' trapped within lymphoid cells present in the tumour rather than the prime cause of the tumour. Recent evidence suggests the possibility that the herpes viruses may act indirectly on cells by activating a latent RNA tumour virus. Ultraviolet light irradiated herpes simplex virus, whilst unable to destroy mouse cells, resulted in the activation of an endogenous virus similar to the RNA tumour viruses.

There is as yet no firm evidence that tumours in humans are caused by viruses; recent work in America suggesting the possible role of a virus as a cause of mammary carcinoma has proved to be ill-founded. The possible involvement of a transmissible viral agent in human sarcomas has been proposed in the last few years. A common surface antigen has been found on sarcoma cells derived from bone, cartilage, fat and muscle and induces a detectable antibody response in patients' serum. This antigen can be transferred to normal human fibroblasts by exposing them to the filtered culture medium from sarcoma cells. That the antigen is transmittable to other individuals is suggested by the finding that cohabitants of sarcoma patients have the anti-sarcoma antibody in their serum.

Carcinomas of the gastrointestinal tract can be shown to contain an antigen absent from normal adult gut cells but present in those of embryos. The antigen termed **carcinoembryonic antigen** (CEA) has been found in the blood of patients with such tumours and their lymphocytes appear to be able to act in vitro against their cultured tumour cells in contrast to control lymphocytes that have no effect.

A somewhat disturbing result of the use of anti-lymphocytic serum (ALS) in man for immunosuppression in tissue transplantation (p. 168) is the small but significantly increased incidence of tumours in such individuals; it seems probable that this is due to suppression of immunological surveillance mechanisms. It is also interesting to note that various chemical immunosuppressive drugs and X-rays, acting like ALS on the lymphoid tissues, are in many instances carcinogens as well as immunosuppressive agents. In recent experiments performed to test the effects of immunosuppression by ALS on tumour incidence, once again the results have not been clear-cut. As in the situation with thymectomized mice, local tumour incidence following chemical carcinogens was increased after ALS treatment. In studies of the development of spontaneous leukaemias in ALS treated mice, there are reports of both increased and decreased tumour incidence and the problem so far remains unresolved.

The incidence of cancer in man is highest at the two extremes of life and it is just at these times that the immune system is least efficient. All these observations point to the probable important role played by the intact mechanisms in keeping the body free of undesirable mutant neoplastic cells.

There is considerable discussion amongst immunologists concerning the particular cells of the immune system that may be responsible for 'surveillance' mechanisms to deal with neoplastic cells or host cells altered in other ways. The emphasis has shifted from a central role for the thymus-dependent (T) lymphocyte (partly because of the conflicting experimental evidence discussed above) to a role for the macrophage which can readily be shown in vitro to have cytotoxic effects against tumour cells (see Fig. 5.7). Tumours are often heavily infiltrated with macrophages, and transfer of such cells in an activated state (see p. 122) to mice with experimental tumours has been shown to lead to tumour suppression. Macrophages undoubtedly have the ability to recognize and bind to their surface (with and without antibody) various foreign materials such as bacteria and altered cells (e.g. red cells), and it is not unreasonable to suppose that this ability might extend to recognition of neoplastic cells.

Tumour antigens
It can be deduced from the foregoing discussion that for the immunological system to react against tumour cells, these cells must

be changed in some way so that they are no longer recognized as self. That this is indeed so is substantiated by many examples of tumours which have been found to develop **new antigens** as part of their cell structure. There are two types of antigenic change: (1) where the specificity of the new antigen is dependent on the inducing agent such as a virus, and (2) tumours induced by chemical carcinogens in which the antigenic change induced by the same carcinogen in two different animals is different in each case. The carcinogen methylcholanthrene has been reported to induce different antigenic changes in cells even in the same animal if the chemical is applied to two separate areas.

There are numerous examples of tumour formation which seem to be associated with these changes. The SV_{40} virus induces tumours in monkeys, the Rous sarcoma virus in chickens and the polyoma virus in mice. The tumours induced in mice by the polyoma virus have recently been shown to consist of two sorts of cells, cells that are malignant on introduction into another mouse and cells that do not survive transplantation. It seems possible that the latter cells are destroyed by the immune system because they carry recognizable foreign antigens on their surface. When cells of the non-transplantable variety are cultured in vitro variants appear which have lost their antigenicity and can thus transfer the tumour. This raises the possibility that attempts to eliminate malignant cells by increasing the immune reaction against them may result in the 'selection' of 'non-antigenic' variants which would allow the tumour to spread.

The tumour-specific antigens are comparable to the weak histocompatibility antigens (p. 161) and their strength has been found to vary for different aetiological groups. Methylcholanthrene-induced sarcomas in mice have been found to be more strongly antigenic than similar sarcomas induced by dibenzanthracene. Among the virus tumours, Moloney virus-induced lymphomas of the mouse are quite strongly antigenic, whereas the Gross agent induces a similar tumour with very weak tumour-specific antigens. Consistent with the finding that the specificity of tumour antigens varies even with one chemical carcinogen is the finding that the strength of these antigens varies also.

Having established that antigenic changes occur in neoplastic cells and that immunological processes are apparently involved in the body's reaction to tumours, the question is, how in fact does any tumour grow and spread throughout the body in the face of the body's immune reaction? Some of the factors which tip the balance in favour of tumour growth have already been discussed in relation to central defects of the immune response.

Another important factor is that the tumour-specific antigens are often not strongly antigenic and the degree of immunity developed is insufficient to cause the rejection of a rapidly growing tumour. In experiments in mice with primary tumours induced by chemical carcinogens, it has been shown that if a mouse is pre-immunized with tumour cells (inactivated by X-irradiation) the animal can then develop a state of immunity to transfer of living tumour cells, provided that the number of transferred cells is not too large to overcome the induced immunity.

The abnormal social behaviour of tumour cells is well known in that they generally fail to form stable intercellular adhesions. It would not be suprising if the interaction between tumour cells and cells of the lymphoid system would likewise be abnormal, leading to escape of the tumour cell from the potentially cytotoxic effects of lymphocytes.

Another way in which tumours could escape the attention of lymphocytes sensitized to the tumour antigens is by the **shedding** from the tumour of excess antigen. Such antigen present in the serum of patients with malignant disease is believed to account for the inhibitory effect of such serum on lymphocyte cytotoxicity for the tumour. Free tumour antigen or antigen-antibody complexes could conceivably 'blindfold' sensitized lymphocytes thus preventing them from identifying and attaching to tumour cells themselves.

Experiments in vitro have shown that complexes of tumour antigen and antibody can interfere with the potentially cytotoxic effects of lymphocytes, presumably by preventing access of the lymphocytes to the tumour cell surface. In a similar way, free tumour antigen can absorb onto the surface of a cytotoxic lymphocyte and be shown to prevent its attaching to the membrane of a tumour cell. The phenomenon in which factors present in the serum block immuces reactions against tumours is known as 'enhancement'. Enhancement does seem to be associated with large progressive tumours. It disappears when the tumour is removed and reappears on recurrence.

In the last few years attention has been directed at the role of T lymphocyte subpopulations (including helper and suppressor cells, p. 43) in the generation of specific cytotoxic cells and antibodies against tumours. The development of suppressor T lymphocytes can be shown in mice when the tumour burden becomes great. Suppression of immune responses in both mice and humans has also been attributed to the activities of B lymphocytes and macrophages.

The immune response against tumour antigens is thus likely to be modified in a variety of ways with consequences that are very difficult to predict. It is likely that a precise understanding of the role of the immune system in tumour immunity will only be gained when the local response at the site of the tumour is analysed. Thus, for example, in the estimation of the role of suppressor T cells, it may be necessary to take into account only those cells in the local tumour environment.

Implications in cancer therapy
The classical treatment for carcinoma of the breast and many other tumours is the radical surgical removal of the neoplastic tissue and much of the surrounding tissue, including the lymph glands of the area.

It is now recognized that this treatment sometimes enhances the spread of secondary deposits, and it is thought that this might be due to removal of lymphoid tissues involved in the immune response to the antigens of the tumour, and possibly also to diminution in the antigenic stimulus to the immune system. The balance is thus tipped in favour of remaining tumour cells which can proliferate unchecked. In addition it should be remembered that mammary carcinogenesis almost certainly also involves the interplay of a variety of non-immunological factors — hormonal, genetic and possibly viral.

A number of ways have been proposed of inhibiting tumour growth by enhancing the immune response to the tumour antigens, either by active immunization with tumour antigens or by non-specifically stimulating the lymphoid tissues. This area is fraught with ethical and practical difficulties but a few partially successful, albeit heroic, experiments have been tried in man.

In one small series in America, malignant tissue was interchanged between pairs of patients with 'incurable' tumours. After allowing sufficient time for an immune response, leucocytes from the immunized individual were injected into the original donor of the tumour tissue. Clinical benefit was claimed in 5 of the 14 patients involved, one patient having complete remission with the disappearance of the numerous secondary tumour deposits of a malignant melanoma with no sign of a recurrence after one year.

Agents known to stimulate the cells of the lymphoid tissues in a non-specific manner have come into vogue in the last few years as a form of cancer immunotherapy. This interest derives from the work in France of Mathé who has employed BCG (p. 140) treatment as part of the therapy of acute lymphoblastic leukaemia in children. The length of the remissions in such cases appeared to be prolonged. The possible value of **non-specific stimulation** of the immune system is pointed to by some recent work with such an agent, *Corynebacterium parvum*. Mice injected with *C. parvum* and given vigorous antitumour chemotherapy showed complete remission in up to 70% of mice with a chemically induced sarcoma. The effect was found only when the two treatments were combined. Other experiments in mice showed that BCG was most effective if given a week or more before the injection of tumour cells. This indicates that the treatment is not likely to be effective in the presence of an established tumour unless some steps are taken to reduce the tumour mass by drug or X-ray therapy.

In tumours of mice associated with vertically transmitted viruses such as the Gross virus, there is no evidence of a specific immune response to virus or tumour and it is assumed that the presence of the virus from early development of the animal leads to immunological tolerance to the virus (see p. 87). Search for a similar situation in human tumours has not been fruitful and histological examination of tumours and associated lymph nodes all point to absence of tolerance.

Non-specific immunodeficiency is often found associated with rapidly growing tumours in humans but it is not clear if this is cause or effect. It appears that patients with early tumours do not usually show lack of immunological competence and that this only appears after fairly extensive tumour growth. This is believed to be due to the appearance of suppressor T lymphocytes and is interpreted to be a consequence of tumour growth rather than a failure of the initial immune surveillance mechanism.

Corynebacterium parvum and BCG injected directly into mouse tumours can be shown dramatically to suppress tumour growth. The effect appears to be largely due to a cell-mediated immune response to the antigens of the microorganisms, in which lymphoid cells are attracted to the injection site in large numbers and appear to act not only on the bacterial antigens but also on the surrounding tumour cells.

Another effect of these organisms is to 'activate' the macrophages of the injected animal in such a way that they can be shown in vitro to become cytotoxic for cultured tumour cells. It is difficult to be sure that this effect operates in vivo but it is possible, at least where tumour cells are circulating in the bloodstream or free in a body cavity, that activated macrophages could capture and destroy them.

In conclusion, it seems possible that immunotherapy may have an important role in the future treatment of malignant disease. It seems likely to be most effective when the tumour mass is small or can be reduced by chemotherapy. The sponteneous disappearance of tumours and complete recovery of patients with widespread cancer does on rare occasions happen and is usually explained as divine intervention. A more readily acceptable explanation of such phenomena is that for some other reason the balance between tumour growth and the immune reaction against it has been tipped in favour of the immune response.

The major difficulty confronting the oncologist in the use of immunotherapy is that there is at present such an incomplete understanding of the relationship of tumours with the immune system that it is not possible to make rational decisions on whether immunotherapy will be of value in any particular situation. Present efforts are initiated largely on an empirical basis that in theory might work but the background knowledge is inadequate to provide a proper scientific basis for treatment. In this situation available resources should clearly be allocated to this end and the attractive option of trying out yet another form of immunotheraphy should be resisted. The history of medical progress, however, is full of examples where empirical observations were found to have real therapeutic value. Nevertheless, it is probably true to say that in most instances they occurred before the recent enormous advances in scientific progress in the cell biological and molecular biological sciences, and that it is no longer justifiable to turn aside from a systematic scientific investigation of a disease state.

FURTHER READING

Bengesh-Melnick M, Batel J S 1974 In: Busch H (ed) The molecular biology of cancer. Academic Press, New York

Burnet F M 1962 The integrity of the body. Oxford University Press, London

Burnet F M 1970 Immunological surveillance. Pergamon Press, London

Chirigos M A 1977 Control of neoplasia by modulation of the immune system. Raven Press, New York

Currie G A 1975 Immunology of malignant disease. In: Bagshawe K D (ed) Medical oncology. Blackwell, Oxford

Currie G A 1980 Cancer and the immune response, 2nd edn. Edward Arnold, London

Fenner F 1968 The pathogenesis and ecology of viral infection. Academic Press, New York

Hamilton Fairley G 1971 Immunity to malignant disease in man. British Journal of Hospital Medicine 6: 633

Lachmann P J, Peters D K (eds) 1982 Clinical aspects of immunology, 4th edn. Blackwell, Oxford

Stutman O 1975 Immunodepression and malignancy. Advances in Cancer Research 22: 261

Trentin J J 1967 Cross-reacting antigens and neo-antigens (with implications for auto-immunity and cancer immunity). Williams and Wilkins, Baltimore

Turk J L 1969 Immunology in clinical medicine. Heinemann, London

9

Immunopathology

Objectives

On completion of this section the reader will be able to:

1. Distinguish between delayed and immediate type hypersensitivity reactions
2. Describe anaphylactic (type 1) reactions and the pharmacological mediators involved
3. Describe cytotoxic (type 2) reactions and antibody-dependent cell-mediated cytotoxicity
4. Describe toxic complex (type 3) reactions and provide two examples
5. Outline the lymphocyte-mediated delayed (type 4) reaction and list two common inducing agents
6. Describe stimulatory (type 5) reactions and list two examples
7. Differentiate the two categories of immunodeficiency state
8. Give three examples of phagocytic defects
9. Give two examples of complement deficiencies and describe their consequences
10. Give two examples of each of the following: primary immunodeficiency state and secondary immunodeficiency state. Describe laboratory procedures for diagnosis of each and available therapies
11. Describe three possible pathogenic mechanisms that might result in autoimmune states
12. Describe the genetic basis of susceptibility to autoimmune diseases
13. Describe the possible role of T cell tolerance in the control of autoantibody producing B cells
14. Provide an example of an autoimmune disease and describe laboratory tests used in its diagnosis.

In the earlier chapters of this section, the immune system has been considered in relation to its role in protection from infection or tumour development and in graft rejection or reaction to transfused blood cells. Such responses can be considered as advantageous to the host in terms of removal of foreign material. As has been noted in Chapter 5, protection is sometimes associated with disadvantageous consequences to the host, as is illustrated by the finding of immune complexes with their effects in the kidneys and elsewhere. In other situations the functioning of the immune system is affected by its exposure to infective agents and in rare instances by inherited defects. In Chapter 4 it was pointed out that in normal individuals self tolerance and the ability to discriminate between self and non-self was an essential feature in the development of the immune system. This ability of the cells of the immune system is not absolute and conditions (largely ill-defined) can arise where self-reactivity, or autoimmunity, occurs. In this chapter an outline is given of these disadvantageous immune responses under the three headings, hypersensitivity, immunodeficiency, and autoimmunity.

HYPERSENSITIVITY

Since immunity was first recognised as a resistant state that followed infection, immunology developed primarily as an aspect of medical bacteriology with emphasis on acquired specific resistance to invasion by microorganisms as a means of protection against infection. Much of the present terminology originates from this early period in the development of immunology. The term immunity, meaning safe or exempt, has now been extended far beyond its early meaning and includes reactions to foreign material such as grafted tissues, blood products and various bland chemical substances none of which bears any relation to infectious agents. Some forms of immune reaction, rather than providing exemption or safety to the affected individual, can produce severe and occasionally fata results. These are known as 'hypersensitivity reactions' and in the main are due to tissue damage caused by effects of pharmacologically active agents such as histamine which are formed under certain conditions of antigen-antibody combination.

The term allergy was originally coined by von Pirquet early this century to describe the altered reactivity of an animal following exposure to a foreign antigen, and included both immunity and hypersensitivity. The term, however, has over the years become restricted to refer only to the hypersensitivity which may be associated with the development of the immune response to a foreign substance.

Immediate and delayed hypersensitivity

There are two main forms of hypersensitivity reaction: **immediate** and **delayed** (Fig. 9.1). The immediate or **antibody-mediated** form appears rapidly and depends on the production of pharmacologically active mediator substances activated by antigen-antibody interaction. The delayed or **cell-mediated** form appears more slowly (usually after 24 hours) and depends on immunologically activated lymphoid cells which, on reaction with antigen, appear to release substances known as lymphokines having a variety of effects on other cells and effects on blood vessel permeability (p. 95).

Fig. 9.1 Hypersensitivity reactions

Various classifications of hypersensitivity reactions have been proposed and probably the most widely accepted is that of Coombs and Gell. This recognises four types or categories of hypersensitivity reactions, three of which come under the heading of immediate antibody-mediated reactions: type 1, anaphylactic reactions; type 2, cytolytic or cytotoxic reactions; and type 3, toxic-complex syndrome. The fourth type is the cell-mediated delayed hypersensitivity form of reaction. An additional category is now recognised that is antibody mediated and can be regarded as a stimulatory form of hypersensitivity. This is sometimes referred to as a type 5 reaction.

Anaphylactic reactions of type 1

If a guinea-pig is injected with a small dose of an antigen such as egg albumen no adverse effects are noted. If however, a second injection of the egg albumen antigen is given intravenously after an interval of about 10 days a condition known as 'anaphylactic shock' is likely to develop. The animal becomes restless, starts chewing and rubbing its nose with its front paws, respiration becomes laboured, the animal becomes cyanosed and may develop convulsions and die. The initial injection of antigen is termed the **sensitising dose** and the second injection the **shocking dose**. During the interval between the two injections the animal has formed antibody. Anaphylaxis is the result of interaction of the shocking dose of antigen with antibody which triggers the release of pharmacologically active substances causing increase in capillary permeability and contraction of smooth muscle in many parts of the body. In the guinea-pig this particularly affects the smooth muscles of the bronchioles, causing respiratory embarrassment.

Pharmacological mediators. Four pharmacologically active substances have been implicated to varying degrees in anaphylactic reactions: (1) histamine, (2) 5-hydroxy-tryptamine, (3) slow-reacting substance, (4) the bradykinins. Predominant amongst these and responsible for many of the symptoms of anaphylactic shock is **histamine** which can be shown to be liberated in vitro when antibody-sensitised pieces of various tissues including uterine muscle, lung and intestine are exposed to contact with antigen. Sensitisation may be produced by prior injection of antigen into the animal supplying the tissue, which makes antibody as described above, or the tissue may be sensitised passively by the addition of antibody produced in another animal. The typical contractions induced in this way in the uterus and intestine are called Schultze-Dale reactions after the originators. The histamine is derived from the granules of mast cells where it exists as its precursor histidine, in combination with heparin; these substances are released by the interaction of antigen with antibody via another pharmacologically active substance, anaphylatoxin, acting together with serum complement components (p. 25). A newly described leucocyte derived group of substances, the leukotrienes, are likely to be important in allergy, and appear to account for the activity of SRS-A.

The eosinophil is thought to play an important part in anaphylactic reactions, many of these marrow-derived cells being found in the blood and tissues during an anaphylactic reaction. Eosinophils are attracted to the site of the reaction by an **eosinophil chemotactic factor** that is released following the interaction of antibody and antigen on the surface of a mast cell. The precise role of the eosinophil in anaphylactic reactions is not yet clear. Its suggested activities include the release of an inhibitor of histamine after having phagocytosed complexes of antibody and antigen and the repair of the tissue damage brought about in the hypersensitivity reaction. Eosinophil granules contain arylsulphatase, an enzyme that splits SRS-A into two inactive fragments and thus can control the smooth muscle spasm induced by SRS-A.

The other pharmacological mediators of immediate hypersensitivity reactions are: 5-hydroxy-tryptamine or serotonin which causes contraction of plain muscle and increased capillary permeability. It is of uncertain role in anaphylaxis, although it is probably involved in local intestinal food allergies; slow-reacting substance (or SRS-A) has a plain muscle contracting effect acting, unlike histamine, on the larger rather than smaller blood vessels. SRS-A has a particularly marked bronchial constricting effect in man and is probably the predominant pharmacological agent in human asthma. Bradykinins are simple peptides formed from a plasma α globulin (kininogen) by plasma kinin-forming enzymes. They have histamine-like effects on smooth muscle and capillaries, and studies have shown that it is present in the bloodstream in many species in the early stages of an anaphylactic reaction.

Systemic and local forms. In man there are two types of anaphylactic reaction — **systemic** and **local** — and which one of these develops depends on how the shocking dose of antigen enters the body. The systemic form of anaphylaxis is likely to develop if antigen is injected parenterally, as in the case of foreign serum (e.g. horse anti-tetanus serum), or a drug such as penicillin, or perhaps by the bite of an insect. The symptoms include dyspnoea with bronchospasm and laryngeal oedema, sometimes skin rashes, a fall in blood pressure and occasionally death. If, on the other hand, the antigen comes in contact with respiratory mucous membranes, then in a sensitised individual the local forms of anaphylaxis will develop — i.e. hay fever or asthma. If the intestinal mucous membrane of a susceptible individual comes in contact with the appropriate antigen (e.g. nuts, fish or strawberries), then a mixed form of reaction can develop with intestinal symptoms, skin rashes (urticaria) and sometimes the symptoms of asthma.

The antibodies involved in anaphylactic reactions

The role of IgE. In the human the antibodies which sensitise the tissues for anaphylactic reactions have been known for many years as **reaginic** antibodies. These antibodies have a strong affinity for tissues (cytotrophic) and can readily be detected in the serum of a sensitised individual by injecting a small quantity of the serum into the skin of a normal recipient, and 24 to 48 hours later, introducing the appropriate antigen into the injection site. Within about 20 minutes a weal and flare erythematous reaction develops at the injection site, just like the response to an injection of histamine. This reaction is called the P.K. test after its originators Prausnitz and Küstner.

The nature of reaginic antibody was not finally elucidated until late in 1967 when a hitherto undescribed form of myeloma protein was discovered in Sweden, although work in America suggested the existence of an immunoglobulin distinct from IgG, IgM or IgA. This made it possible (using an antiserum to the myeloma globulin prepared in a sheep) to show in normal human serum a new class of immunoglobulin present in very low concentration (10–130 μg/ 100 ml of serum cf. 900–1800 mg of IgG/100 ml serum). The skin-sensitising activity of reaginic antibody could readily be neutralised by means of the antiserum to this new immunoglobulin which has been named IgE (p. 134). The concentration of IgE in patients with allergic asthma has been found to be much higher than in normal individuals although the level of IgE in the circulation does not correlate with the severity of the allergic symptoms. The comparatively low levels of IgE found in serum presumably reflect the affinity of this immunoglobulin for tissues so that freshly made IgE is very soon removed from serum when it comes in contact with the appropriate cell receptors on mast cells and possibly elsewhere.

IgE appears to have four main activities: (1) the capacity to bind via its Fc fragment to mast cells in basophils; (2) subsequent interaction with antigen that takes place on the cell membrane of the mast cell; (3) resultant triggering of the release of pharmacological mediators; (4) attraction of other cell types — eosinophils. The third of these activities, namely the triggering of the release of pharmacological mediators from mast cells, has been the subject of much recent study and it appears that two adjacent molecules of IgE (attached to Fc receptors on mast cells) must be **bridged** by antigen before degranulation takes place. Monovalent antigens (i.e., with a single antigenic determinant) will block the IgE antibody from further interaction with antigen but will **not** trigger degranulation. The triggering appears to follow the entry of calcium ions into the mast cell, presumably as part of the membrane changes that finally lead to the degranulation or exocytosis process.

Immunological approaches to the prevention of anaphylaxis

Blocking antibody. On consideration of the mechanism of systemic anaphylaxis it would seem likely that if the parenterally injected antigen could be prevented from reaching the tissue-fixed IgE then anaphylaxis would not develop. This desirable state of affairs can be achieved by the simple expedient of injecting frequent small doses of the antigen to which the patient is sensitised. This induces the formation of increasing levels of IgG antibody which, circulating in the blood and tissue fluids, mops up the in-

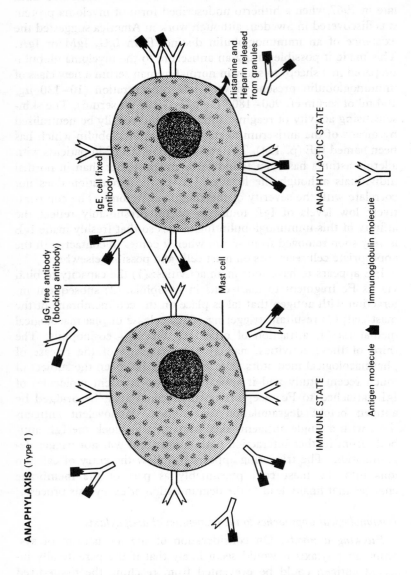

Fig. 9.2 Diagrammatic view of the possible difference between an *'immune state'* (i.e. when immunised animal will not develop anaphylaxis on challenge with antigen) and an *'anaphylactic state'*. Here there is insufficient antibody free in the tissue fluids to mop up the antigen thus allowing it to combine with reaginic antibody (IgE) attached to cell. The interaction triggers the release of histamine and heparin from mast cell granules.

jected antigen so that it does not reach the tissue-fixed IgE (Fig. 9.2). This IgG antibody has been termed **blocking antibody** and its induction is the basis of desensitisation treatment in allergic individuals. As might be expected this method is much more effective in preventing systemic anaphylactic reactions than the local forms where the antigen does not enter the bloodstream. To prevent local anaphylaxis the blocking antibody would need to be present in the mucous secretions and parenteral injection of antigen is hardly the best way to achieve this (see p. 124 for discussion of immunisation against influenza virus).

In theory it should be possible, by raising the level of IgE to antigens other than those responsible for the allergic sensitisation, to occupy the tissue receptors by non-specific IgE antibodies rather than those formed to the sensitising antigen. Whether such a procedure is feasible remains to be established. Recent work using rats sensitised to benzylpenicilloyl (a penicillin derivative) raises the possibility that B cell tolerance can be induced to the antigen by repeated injections (subcutaneously or intraperitoneally) of the benzylpenicilloyl linked to a carrier, a random polymer of glutamic acid and lysine (D–GL). Levels of IgE and IgG to the penicillin derivative are markedly reduced for at least six months.

For pollen or seasonal allergies, desensitising injections are given before the onset of the pollen season. About 70% of cases obtain clinical benefit from the treatment, and with ragweed antigen marked increases in the ratio of blocking IgG to IgE levels have recently been found.

Symptomatic treatment of allergies commonly involves the use of anti-histamines and more recently disodium cromoglycate has come into use. This is effective in blocking histamine release if the drug is present before challenge with antigen. Isoprenaline and theophylline, which increase the level of intracellular cyclic-AMP, in turn reduce histamine release from mast cells. Corticosteroids also have a beneficial effect in type 1 allergic disorders, although their mode of action is unclear.

Cytolytic or cytotoxic (type 2) reactions

Cell-associated antigens. Reactions of this type are initiated by an antigenic component either part of a tissue cell or closely associated with it (e.g. a drug attached to the cell wall (Fig. 9.3). The antibodies directed against such a cell-associated antigen bring about a cytotoxic or cytolytic effect usually involving complement. Reactions of this type include the cytolytic effect of anti-red cell antibodies, induced by incompatible blood transfusion, on the foreign

Fig. 9.3 Cytolytic and cytotoxic (type 2) reactions

erythrocytes. Haemolytic disease of the newborn has a similar mechanism as do certain forms of auto-immune haemolytic anaemia in which the patient forms antibodies against autologous red cells.

There are many examples of these cytotoxic or cytolytic reactions which are brought about by an immune reaction to a foreign substance attached to the cell membranes of erythrocytes, leucocytes or platelets. One of the best known examples of this phenomenon is Sedormid (apronal) purpura. The complexing of the drug Sedormid with platelets results in an antibody response directed against the platelet-adsorbed drug which brings about destruction of the platelets and purpura. As a result of the elucidation of the mechanism of this disease by Ackroyd in London, Sedormid has been withdrawn from use. This type of reaction may be more widespread than is generally suspected. A variety of infectious diseases due to salmonella organisms and mycobacteria are associated with haemolytic anaemia, and there is evidence, particularly in studies in salmonella infections, that the haemolysis is due to an immune reaction against a lipopolysaccharide bacterial endotoxin which becomes coated on to the patient's erythrocytes. A detailed study of *Salmonella gallinarum* infection in chickens has shown conclusively that the red cells are coated, have a shorter life in the circulation due to haemolysis, and that the development of haemolysis directly parallels the level of the anti-lipopolysaccharide antibody.

Antibody-dependent cell-mediated cytotoxicity

This mixed form of hypersensitivity is mediated by at least two distinct types of non-immune cells acting in conjunction with antibody directed at a target cell.

The non-immune 'killer' cells (or K cells) take two forms:

1. Cells morphologically similar to small or medium-sized lymphocytes without easily demonstrable immunoglobulin on their surface that are not glass adherent (in contrast to macrophages) or phagocytic. They are prominent in human peripheral blood and have receptors for the Fc portion of IgG and sometimes for products of C3. It is believed that these cells are cytotoxic for antibody coated tumour cells (e.g. melanoma cells) and for virus infected cells (e.g. herpes simplex infected cells).

2. A glass adherent cell (possibly a monocyte) that lyses antibody coated red blood cells. This form of lysis takes place without involving the complement system.

These mixed forms of hypersensitivity reaction can readily be demonstrated in vitro and there a number of reports showing cytotoxic effects against various antibody-coated target cells including human tissue cells in certain 'auto-immune' disease states (see Ch. 9). Whether or not this mixed form of hypersensitivity has its in vivo counterpart remains to be established.

In these reactions, damage to cells is the result of the attachment of antibody to their surface. The consequences include (see Fig. 9.4):

1. direct lysis of the cells by complement activation

2. adherence to phagocytes by their Fc and C3 receptors leading to phagocytosis

3. antibody-dependent cell-mediated cytotoxicity (ADCC), by both phagocytic and non-phagocytic cells (PMNs and macrophages) and cells morphologically similar to lymphocytes but with Fc receptors, referred to as K cells.

The cytotoxic effects require contact between the effector and target cell and is independent of complement components.

The situations where such cytotoxic reactions develop are the result of the expression of antigen on the surface of a cell that leads to antibody production. Such antigen expression can be initiated in a variety of ways (Fig. 9.4) as already indicated.

Fig. 9.4 Type II antibody-dependent cytotoxic hypersensitivity

Toxic-complex syndrome (type 3) reactions

Serum sickness and Arthus reactions. These reactions are due to the combination of antigen with circulating antibody, with the formation of microprecipitates in and around small blood vessels. This causes inflammation and sometimes mechanical blocking of these vessels which results in interference with the blood supply to surrounding tissues. There are two types of reaction which fall into this category: **serum sickness** which is a systemic form and the **Arthus reaction** which is a local form.

Serum sickness develops, as the name suggests, in individuals injected with foreign serum and was described soon after the introduction of parenteral administration, for therapeutic purposes, of diphtheria antitoxin prepared in the horse. Foreign serum protein is eliminated from the circulation over a period of a few weeks and after the injection of 10 to 20 ml there will still be a large amount present by the time an immune response to the foreign serum protein develops. This results in the formation of antibody-antigen complexes that can cause a wide variety of symptoms ranging from anaphylactic reactions such as asthma or laryngeal oedema when IgE antibody attached to mast cells is involved, to symptoms dependent on the deposition of immune complexes (antigen + IgG antibody) in blood vessels where they activate complement and cause inflammatory changes. Fixation of the first component of complement (p. 25) leads to the formation of anaphylatoxin involved in histamine release. The inflammatory cells are mainly polymorphs attracted by the trimolar C567 complex that has chemotactic activity. Proteolytic enzymes released by polymorphs damage adjacent tissues and plasma kinins are also activated. The intensity of the reaction depends upon the concentration of complexes and on the ability of the antibody to activate complement.

IgM, IgG1, IgG2 and IgG3 antibodies have this ability (p. 72) whereas IgG4, IgA and IgE do not. The clinical manifestations depend upon where the immune complexes form or lodge.

On the basis of experimental work in rabbits two forms of reaction have been recognised: (1) following a single large dose of antigen which results in arthritis, glomerulonephritis and coronary artery vasculitis; (2) following daily doses of antigen which results after a few weeks in glomerulonephritis. The first form is complement-dependent whereas the second occurs even in complement-depleted animals. The first form of reaction in humans manifests itself by affecting the kidneys with the development of glomerulonephritis and in severe cases renal failure, the heart, with myocarditis and valvulitis, and the joints which become swollen and painful. Urticaria sometimes develops and the patient becomes pyrexial. The symptoms disappear whenever all the foreign serum protein is eliminated.

Antigens other than serum proteins can cause serum sickness. Nowadays the most likely causes are drugs such as penicillin and sulphonamides. The susceptible patient will develop rashes (urticarial, morbilliform or scarlatinoform), pyrexia, arthralgia, lymphadenopathy and perhaps nephritis some 8 to 12 days after being given the drug. It seems likely that many bacterial infections, and some virus ones, include development of hypersensitivity of this type, as rashes, joint pains and sometimes mild haematuria are not uncommon (see Fig. 9.5). In post-streptococcal glomerulonephritis streptococcal antigens have been detected in the glomeruli (see

Fig. 9.5 Type III Immune complex hypersensitivity — causes and consequences

also p. 206). In virus hepatitis circulating immune complexes have been found associated with periarteritis nodosa. Many of the clinical features of the autoimmune disease systemic lupus erythematosus (discussed on p. 208) appear to result from arteritis, and deposits of immunoglobulin and complement (probably complexed with DNA) have been found in the skin lesions and glomeruli of patients with the disease.

The Arthus reaction, like serum sickness, is brought about by the formation of antibody-antigen complexes but in this case the phenomenon is a local one at the site of injection of antigen. The Arthus reaction occurs in walls of small blood vessels in the presence of large quantities of IgG antibody forming microprecipitates with antigen. The resulting vasculitis develops a few hours after injection of antigen and persists for 12 to 24 hours. Immune complexes can be shown microscopically in the vessel wall using the fluorescent antibody technique (p. 233) and there is a massive infiltration of granulocytes brought about by a chemotactic effect generated by the antigen-antibody complex. There is activation of the vasoactive amines such as histamine, with resulting increase in vascular permeability and consequent oedema. These reactions may occur in diabetics who have received many injections of insulin and have developed high levels of IgG antibody to antigenic constituents in the insulin preparation.

Arthus reactions in the bronchial or alveolar wall may explain the late asthmatic reactions that occur 7 to 8 hours after inhalation of antigen. These may be of particular importance in the 'allergic alveolitis' seen in farmers sensitive to mouldy hay antigen (see p. 136) and maltworkers sensitive to *Aspergillus clavatus* of contaminated barley. In some cases of tuberculosis, sarcoidosis, leprosy and streptococcal infections, vascular inflammatory lesions are seen mainly in the legs. These are variously referred to as erythema nodosum, nodular vasculitis and erythema induratum and may be due to the deposition of immune complexes and the development of an Arthus reaction.

Delayed hypersensitivity (type 4) cell-mediated hypersensitivity

Lymphocyte-mediated reactions and 'lymphokines'. These can be defined as specifically provoked, slowly evolving (24 to 48 hours), mixed cellular reactions involving lymphocytes and macrophages. The reaction is not brought about by circulating antibody but by sensitised lymphoid cells and can be transferred in experimental animals by means of such cells but not serum. The classical example of this type of reaction is the tuberculin response which has over the years received detailed study. To induce this response a tuberculin-sensitised individual is given an intradermal injection of 0.1 ml of a 1 in 1000 dilution of a protein extract of tubercle bacilli (purified protein derivative PPD). An indurated inflammatory reaction in the skin, measuring a few millimetres in diameter, appears about 24 hours later and persists for a few weeks. In the human the injection site is infiltrated with large numbers of mononuclear cells, mainly lymphocytes, with about 10–20% macrophages. Most of these cells are in and around small blood vessels.

Despite intensive investigation of the delayed hypersensitivity reaction, immunologists are far from understanding the mechanisms underlying this phenomenon. A possible explanation is that amongst the continuous traffic of lymphocytes passing through the tissues (p. 96) there are some sensitised cells, possibly with 'antibody-like receptors' on their surface. These cells interact with antigen they meet and in some unknown way influence other lymphocytes and phagocytes to migrate to the area (see also Table 4.1).

In the last few years a group of as yet ill-defined substances have been shown to be released by lymphocytes coming in contact with the antigen to which they have been sensitised. The name **lymphokines** has been proposed to describe this group of non-antibody lymphocyte factors. They are discussed on page 92 and Table 4.6 shows the range of factors produced. Their main role appears to be to **recruit** non-sensitised (uncommitted) lymphoid cells to the site of inflammation and to **retain** them at the site where they become activated, thus **amplifying** the immune response. An important factor appears to be responsible for inducing proliferation of lymphocytes at the site of localisation and has been termed mitogenic factor. A cytotoxic effect has been demonstrated in tissue culture experiments affecting lymphocytes and other cells (lymphotoxin).

The best known of the lymphokines is the macrophage migration inhibition factor. This effect is readily demonstrated in vitro using peritoneal exudate cells from an animal sensitised to an antigen such as tuberculin. The peritoneal exudate cells, which are mainly macrophages, are collected in a capillary tube that is placed on a glass coverslip in a small tissue culture chamber (Fig. 4.23). After 24 hours macrophages show a fan-shaped area of migration around the end of the capillary tube. If, however, the tuberculin antigen is placed in the tissue culture medium no migration occurs. The effect appears to be due to the release, from the small number of lymphocytes in peritoneal exudate, of a lymphokine known as macrophage migration inhibition factor or MIF. The specificity of the reaction has been shown with several other antigens including bovine gamma globulin, histoplasmin and dinitrophenol. The MIF appears to be released from cells concerned with the cell-mediated immune state rather than cells concerned with making humoral antibody.

The chemical nature of MIF has not yet been established although it appears in guinea pigs to have an MW of 35–50 000 (like some of the other lymphokines) and is likely to be glycoprotein. In vivo the factor may be responsible for the formation of large aggregates of macrophages in the lymphoid tissues (and perhaps elsewhere), although like the other lymphokines the precise role of MIF in delayed hypersensitivity reactions is not yet clear. Much further work is required to separate and identify the nature and functional activities of the various substances involved. Whether or not macrophages in delayed hypersensitivity reaction sites contribute lysosomal enzymes from their intracellular granules, thus bringing about further inflammatory changes, has yet to be determined.

Inducing agents. Delayed hypersensitivity reactions are characteristically induced by intracellular infectious agents including salmonellae, brucellae, streptococci and a wide range of viruses including measles and mumps viruses, vaccinia and herpes simplex (see also p. 127). Those with most clinical relevance are reactions due to vaccinia — the so-called 'reaction of immunity' occurring 24 to 72 hours after vaccination. This reaction does not proceed like a primary vaccination through the pustular stage and leaves no scar but instead has all the features of a delayed hypersensitivity reaction. The other important reaction is the 'pseudo-Schick' response occurring within 24 hours after the intradermal injection of diphtheria toxoid. This delayed response disappears within 6 days and also affects the control injected site (heat-treated toxoid).

Delayed hypersensitivity reactions sometimes develop following sensitisation to a variety of metals such as nickel and chromium, to simple chemical substances such as dyestuffs, potassium dichromate (affecting cement workers), primulin from primula plants, poison ivy and chemicals such as picryl chloride, dinitrochlorobenzene, and paraphenylene diamine (from hair dyes). Penicillin sensitisation is a common clinical complication following the tropical application of the antibiotic in ointments or creams. These substances are not themselves antigenic and only become so on combination by covalent bonds with proteins in the skin. The clinical symptoms induced in these 'contact hypersensitivity' reactions (contact dermatitis) include redness, swelling, vesicles, scaling and exudation of fluid.

It is conceivable that, in future, use may be made of the delayed hypersensitivity response in the treatment of tumours. Some recent experiments in man show that certain skin tumours, if painted with a simple chemical antigen as described above, underwent a marked hypersensitivity reaction and then healed with the disappearance of the tumour. One explanation of the effect is that the lymphokine — lymphotoxin — is released during the hypersensitivity reaction and destroys the tumour cells. Much more work is clearly required before this can be regarded as a useful clinical procedure (see also p. 177).

Stimulatory hypersensitivity type V
Non-complement activating antibodies in certain situations can actually stimulate rather than destroy tissue cells. In such situations, the stimulus can be disadvantageous as when an autoantibody — thyroid stimulating antibody — is produced in thyrotoxic patients and produces the same effect as thyroid stimulating hormone activating adenyl cyclase in the membrane that generates cyclic — AMP from ATP with resulting stimulation of thyroid cell activity. Not all antibodies that bind to TSH receptors increase the synthesis of thyroid hormones and some may block access to the receptor of TSH and could theoretically be a cause of hypothyroidism.

IMMUNODEFICIENCY STATES

The immunologically competent cells of the lymphoid tissues derived from, renewed and influenced by the activity of the thymus, bone marrow and probably gut-associated lymphoid tissues, can be the subject of disease processes due either to defects in one of the components of the complex itself, or secondarily to some other disease process affecting the normal functioning of some part of the lymphoid tissues. In 1953 Bruton first described hypogammaglobulinaemia in an 8-year-old boy who developed septic arthritis of the knee at 4 years of age followed by numerous attacks of otitis media, pneumococcal sepsis and pneumonia. Electrophoretic analysis of the serum proteins showed almost complete absence of the gammaglobulin fraction. The child appeared unable to give an immune response to typhoid and diphtheria immunisation. It is now recognised that this form of deficiency is only one of a group of specific deficiencies affecting the lymphoid tissues which can affect both sexes, manifest themselves at any age and be genetically determined or arise secondarily to some other condition.

Before considering specific defects in the acquired immune

response there are a small number of defects that need to be considered in the innate immune mechanisms that possibly involve defects in phagocyte function.

Defective innate immune mechanisms

Defects in phagocytic function take two forms, (1) Where there is a **quantitative** deficiency of blood leucocytes which may be **congenital** (e.g. infantile agranulocytosis) or **acquired** as a result of replacement of bone marrow by tumour tissue or the toxic effects of chemicals. (2) Where there is a **qualitative** deficiency in the functioning of neutrophil leucocytes which, whilst ingesting bacteria normally, fail, because of an enzymic defect, to digest them. The clinical form of this defect is known as chronic granulomatous disease and is a sex-linked recessive condition characterised by increased susceptibility to infection in early life by microorganisms of low virulence to the normal individual. In this condition the monocytes and polymorphs fail to produce H_2O_2 due to a defect in the hexose monophosphate shunt nicotinamide adenine dinucleotide phosphate (NADPH) pathway that is normally activated by phagocytosis (see p. 20). Phagocyte enzyme defects can be detected by the NBT test (p. 246). The ability of the patient's phagocytes to kill bacteria to which they are insusceptible is much reduced and organisms can survive for 2 hours or more within the phagocyte.

Other enzyme defects include deficiency of white blood cell glucose 6-phosphate dehydrogenase. In such patients the NBT test may be normal, but the intracellular activity of the phagocytes is reduced. Hydrogen peroxidase deficiency has also been described. This enzyme is necessary for normal intracellular killing, but the phagocytes from patients with this defect also show normal NBT tests.

Defects in the ability of phagocytes to respond to chemotactic stimuli have been described. Such defects include the lazy leucocyte syndrome and Chediak-Higashi syndrome, the latter condition being a multisystem disorder characterised by giant cytoplasmic inclusions in white blood cells and platelets. In this condition the lysosomal granules are structurally and functionally abnormal, and there is an associated reduction in intracellular killing of microorganisms.

The complement system (p. 24) can also suffer from certain defects in function leading to increased susceptibility to infection. The defects that have been described include: C1q deficiency, C1r and C1s deficiency, C2, C3, C6, C7, C8 deficiency, and dysfunction of the C5 component. Many of these disorders, which are very rare,

are associated with an increased incidence of autoimmune disease (p. 201).

The most severe abnormalities of host defences occur, as would be expected, if there is a defect in the functioning of C3. Severe deficiency or absence of C3 is associated with increased susceptibility to infection, particularly pneumonia, meningitis, otitis, and pharyngitis. Individuals with inherited C3 deficiency can be shown to have normal C1, C4, and C2 activation. Activation of the alternate pathway or components C5–C9 does not occur. Thus normal chemotactic (C5a) and leucocytosis promoting factors (C3e) are absent.

Individuals with C1, C4, and C2 deficiencies tend not to be particularly susceptible to infections due to their intact alternate pathway mechanisms. C5 dysfunction may lead to deficient phagocyte activity with associated recurrent infections and C6, C7, and C8 deficiency with inability to lyse susceptible bacteria such as *Neisseria*, *Salmonella*, and *Haemophilus* organisms.

Diseases in which defects in complement components occur include sickle cell disease and systemic lupus erythematosus (SLE). In sickle cell disease (red cells contain abnormal haemoglobin) there appears to be a defect involving the alternate pathway, and in SLE there is a reduction in levels of the C4 component, sometimes in the C2 component. In addition, persons with SLE appear to have a specific inhibitor of C5-derived chemotactic activity, with the associated susceptibility to infection.

Primary defects
In the first category are the congenital defects affecting immunoglobulin synthetic mechanisms, cell-mediated immune mechanisms or sometimes both. Deficiency of immunoglobulin synthesis is complete in Bruton type agammaglobulinaemia, an X-linked recessive character found in boys and in which the IgG level is reduced by about a tenth and the IgA and IgM about a hundredth of normal values. Cell-mediated immune mechanisms function normally in these patients, who can reject grafts and develop normal delayed hypersensitivity to tuberculosis. However, they do not give the normal circulating antibody response to bacterial vaccines and are thus very susceptible to pyogenic infections. The lymphoid tissue in the appendix and Peyer's patches is somewhat reduced, and patients do not develop plasma cells and germinal centres in lymph nodes.

Partial defects in immunoglobulin synthesis have been described affecting one or more of the main immunoglobulin classes. For example (a) the IgG or IgA levels may be reduced and the IgM level raised; (b) the IgA and IgM may be reduced and the IgG level be normal or (c) the IgA level may be reduced and the others normal.

Electrophoresis of serum as shown in Figure 9.6 cannot distinguish between the various immunoglobulin deficiencies and will only show gross changes in total immunoglobulins. Gel diffusion and immunoelectrophoretic techniques (p. 225) using anti-immunoglobulin antisera are required for the detailed analysis of these deficiencies.

In (a), which is inherited as an X-linked recessive character, the lymphoid tissues appear normal histologically although the plasma cells appear to be making predominantly IgM. Patients are susceptible to pyogenic infectious and the condition is often associated with anaemia, thrombocytopoenia and neutropenia. In (b) even the IgG which is produced in normal quantity is thought to be abnormal in some way and unable to combine with antigen. Defect (c) occurs in 80% of patients with a condition known as hereditary ataxia telangiectasia who have increased susceptibility to infections of the upper and lower respiratory tract. There is a deficiency in plasma cells in the mucous membranes of the intestinal tract, where IgA is known to be produced in normal individuals, and the disease

Fig. 9.6 Tracings obtained by ultraviolet scanning of electrophoretic patterns of human sera. (1) normal serum (2) reduced gamma globulin (antibody deficiency syndrome possible B cell defect) (3) raised gamma globulin (possible myeloma). Peaks right to left: albumin, alpha, beta and gamma globulins (see Fig. 4.13)

seems likely to be due to lack of protection at the level of the respiratory mucous membranes normally brought about by IgA secretion.

Both **cell-mediated** immune mechanisms and **immunoglobulin synthesis** are deficient in an X-linked disease of male children known as 'Swiss-type agammaglobulinaemia' or severe combined immunodeficiency. There is almost complete absence of lymphoid tissue in the body, the thymus is very small and the lymphoid tissues of the appendix and Peyer's patches are absent. Children with this condition cannot make antibodies or develop cell-mediated immune reactions, and they suffer from progressive bacterial and/or viral infection and die within two years of birth.

In another type of deficiency state only the cell-mediated immune mechanisms are affected and there is thymic dysplasia and deficiency of lymphoid cells from those areas of the spleen and lymph nodes which are under thymic control. Although children with this rare type of deficiency can produce circulating antibody, their inability to develop cell-mediated immunity renders them highly susceptible to virus infection. One form of this condition associated with thymic dysplasia and absence of parathyroid glands is known as Di George's syndrome.

Secondary defects
Acquired deficiencies of the immunological mechanisms can occur secondarily to a number of disease states affecting the lymphoid tissues, such as Hodgkin's disease, multiple myeloma, leukaemia and lymphosarcoma. Deficiency of immunoglobulins can also be brought about by excessive loss of protein through diseased kidneys or via the intestines in protein-losing enteropathy. Malnutrition and iron deficiency can lead depressed immune responsiveness, particularly in cell-mediated immunity. Viral infections can be immunosuppressive. For example, measles and other viruses infect cells of the immune system (p. 128). Medical and surgical treatment such as X-rays, cytotoxic drugs, steroids and catheterisation can lead to the state referred to as the 'compromised host' in which there is interference with the effectiveness of the innate and acquired immune mechanisms.

In contrast to the deficiency states just described, raised immunoglobulin levels are found in certain disorders of plasma cell function, which amount to malignant proliferation of a particular clone or family of plasma cells. In this condition, known as multiple myeloma, a malignant clone is found to produce one particular class of immunoglobulin, usually IgG or more rarely one of the other classes. The frequency of occurrence among myeloma of particular immunoglobulin classes reflects their relative levels in serum. There is usually a decreased synthesis of normal immuno-globulins associated with a deficient immune response to infective agents. On electrophoresis of serum a distinct band can be seen in the immunoglobulin area, and Figure 9.6 shows an example of the type of pattern found on simple paper electrophoresis. This abnor-mal band is produced by the raised levels of the myeloma im-munoglobulin which is termed an M-type protein. In about 20 to 30% of patients with multiple myeloma immunoglobulin light chains are found in the urine. These occur as dimers and are known as Bence-Jones protein. The condition is also associated with excess numbers of plasma cells in the bone marrow and X-ray evidence of myeloma cell deposits in bone.

Clinical aspects

Increased susceptibility to many types of infection is the outstand-ing feature of the immunological deficiency states. The age of onset of the congenital types is rarely earlier than 3 to 4 months of age due to the protective effects of maternal antibody. The most frequently affected site is the respiratory tract, which is attacked by pyogenic bacteria or fungi. Lack of IgA antibody leads to particular suscepti-bility to chronic infection of the respiratory tract. Other clinical features frequently associated with immune deficiency states are skin rashes, diarrhoea, growth failure, enlarged liver and spleen and recurrent abscesses or osteomyelitis.

When there is deficiency of the cell-mediated immune mechan-isms, resistance to virus infections is diminished and may be recog-nised by the severe necrosis that will occur at the site of smallpox vaccination. BCG vaccination can lead to generalised tuberculosis infection in such cases.

Investigation of suspected immunological deficiency states should include family studies for any abnormalities of immune function. Lymphocyte function may be assessed by stimulation (a) with non-specific agents such as PHA or concanavalin A (p. 245) or (b) with a specific bacterial antigen in subjects previously sensitised to the bacterial antigen by natural infection or immunisation (e.g. the tubercle bacillus). Quantitative determination of immunoglobulin levels can be made (p. 244) and estimation of the response to im-munisation with standard antigens. Peripheral blood counts and X-rays of the thymus region may also prove useful.

Treatment of deficiency states includes use of an appropriate antibiotic and regular administration of pooled human immunoglo-bulins. Closely matched sibling bone marrow has been used suc-

Fig. 9.7 Primary immunodeficiency and the cells of the immune system

cessfully in some cases and a graft of fetal thymus has been used in the case of thymic aplasia. Bone marrow grafts can be rejected in the same way as other grafts (Ch. 7) unless closely related to the recipient. An additional complication arises in that the graft may attack host cells — a graft versus host (GVH) reaction (p. 172). In immune deficiency states graft rejection is likely to be the lesser of the two problems. Total lymph node irradiation has been found to be preferable to whole-body irradiation in the control of GVH reactions. Pluripotent stem cells (p. 40) of the bone marrow are likely to become tolerant to host antigens and give rise to mature cells that will not react against host cells. This can be made use of as techniques using monoclonal antibodies come into use to separate various subpopulations within the bone marrow. Figure 9.7 shows the components of the immune system with examples of deficiencies affecting them indicating the effects and possible forms of treatment.

AUTOIMMUNITY

A fundamental characteristic of an animal's immune system is that it does not under normal circumstances react against its own body constituents. There exists a mechanism which enables the cells of the immune system to recognise what is '**foreign**' and what is '**self**'. Attempts to explain the absence of reactions against self go back to the early days of immunology when Paul Ehrlich enunciated his well known doctrine of 'horror autotoxicus'. Ehrlich and Morgenroth in 1900, after immunising a goat with red blood cells of other goats, found that although the animal readily made antibodies against the red cells of other goats these antibodies failed to react with the animal's own red cells. It was thus clear that in some way the immunological response to self antigens was prevented. So powerful was the influence of Paul Ehrlich that it seemed inconceivable that in any circumstances the rule could be broken so that an immunological reaction against self could develop. The view continued to be held despite clinical evidence indicating that diseases existed in which the patient was apparently destroying his own cells.

The main reason that observations of this type failed to achieve the recognition they deserved was the absence of serological techniques capable of demonstrating convincingly the existence of antibodies able to react with tissue cells, or of the presence of such antibodies actually attached to cells. It was not until 1945 that immunologists were provided with this vital tool, when Coombs, Mourant and Race described a technique which detected the presence of antibody globulin on red blood cells by the simple expedient of adding an antiserum against human globulin which, after reacting with the globulin coating the cells, linked the cells together and agglutinated them. This method was particularly valuable for showing antibody globulin adsorbed to cells which was in itself unable to agglutinate the cells.

This technique is commonly known as the 'Coombs' or 'antiglobulin' test (p. 231). The development of the antiglobulin techniques led to the use of antiglobulin sera in a variety of different ways, many of which involved complicated technical operations but which essentially were based on the original antiglobulin method. Amongst the most important of the developments of the method is the fluorescent antibody technique in which one of the most commonly used procedures is to label an antiglobulin serum with a fluorescent marker (fluorescein isothiocyanate) so that the reaction of the labelled antiglobulin with, for example, globulin-coated cells can be visualised under UV light microscopy. Under these conditions the sites of attachment of the fluorescein-labelled antiglobulin show up as bright apple-green fluorescent areas (p. 233).

The recognition of autoimmune disease
These methods allowed a breakthrough in the recognition of a variety of human and animal diseases in which antibodies could be convincingly demonstrated in serum capable of reacting with a number of different antigens of the individual's own tissues.

The first of these was the demonstration that in some types of haemolytic anaemia in man the red blood cells were coated with antibody globulin. This was soon followed by the finding of an autoantibody serum factor in the blood of patients with a severe connective tissue disease called systemic lupus erythematosus (SLE). This factor appeared to be antibody against the nuclei of tissue cells and was called by the author and his colleagues antinuclear factor (ANF). At the same time, workers interested in diseases of the thyroid gland demonstrated the presence of an antibody to thyroglobulin in patients with a particular form of interstitial thyroiditis known as Hashimoto's disease.

The first recognisable clinical description of acquired haemolytic anaemia was given in 1898 in France, and in 1908 haemolytic activity against red cells was found in the serum of patients in whom intense haemolysis was taking place in vivo. These early observations were neglected until 30 years later when Damashek and Schwartz again reported haemolysins in patients suffering from haemolytic anaemia, and with the introduction of the Coombs test in 1945 the immunological basis of the disease was put on a firm foundation.

The effect on immunological theory
Associated with the accumulating evidence on the autoimmune nature of the haemolysins in acute haemolytic anaemia, there arose the need to consider the meaning of foreignness and self-recognition and the mechanisms underlying the ability of the body to differentiate between 'self' and 'non-self'. A solution to the problem this created in immunological theory was offered by Burnet and Fenner in 1949. At that time antibody production was envisaged in terms of the antigen acting as a template for modifying the globulin molecules to a form which was complementary to that of antigen (p. 86). It was considered that antigen might act either on the already formed protein chain and bring about a reconfiguration of the chain, or that the antigen induced a chemical rearrangement of the globulin molecule as it was formed.

Burnet and Fenner, whilst accepting this direct template theory, included the notion of 'self-markers' attached to body components by which antibody-forming cells were able to recognise them, rendering them immunologically inert. They also predicted that an equivalent tolerance to foreign antigens should be demonstrable if these had been introduced at an appropriate stage in embryonic life, while the animal's immune system was in the process of learning to recognise the 'self-markers' of its own tissues. This prediction was later confirmed experimentally by Medawar and his colleagues who showed that if neonatal mice were injected with transplantation antigen from another strain of mice, they would later be able to accept skin grafts which an animal not injected neonatally would rapidly reject.

Burnet soon followed his 'self-marker' theory by his rather more plausible '**clonal selection**' theory. This allowed the antigen no part in impressing a pattern on the antibody-producing cells. The capacity to produce a given antibody was regarded as a genetically determined quality of certain clones or families of mesenchymal cells, the function of the antigen being to stimulate cells of these clones to proliferation and antibody production. The theory postulated that in the early stages of embryonic development, mutation of cells led to a variety of **random** arrangements in the globulin molecules so that a very large number of clones were generated which could correspond to potential antigenic determinants (p. 90). To explain the inability of the antibody-forming system to react with self, Burnet proposed that the immature cells could be destroyed if they came across the antigens with which they could react at this early stage. Whenever the antigenic determinants were freely present in the body and accessible to the corresponding immunologically competent cells, such destructive contacts would be inevitable. Tolerance would result from the elimination or inhibition of all cells clones which had the ability to react with antigenic determinants present in the body. After birth, when foreign antigen entered the tissues, antibody to it would be produced by specific stimulation of those cells in clones preadapted to react with the corresponding antigenic determinants. On the basis of this theory Burnet accounted for the development of autoimmune disease as a failure of the destruction of the self-reactive population of antibody-forming cells (see also p. 87).

Possible mechanisms involved in the development of autoimmunity

The question now arises of how the normal controlling mechanism fails with the resulting inability to maintain self-recognition manifested by immune reactions against self.

There are three main ways (Table 9.1) in which this tolerance-maintaining mechanism could conceivably be overcome. The first involves evasion or circumvention of a normally functioning mechanism and the second failure of the mechanism itself. The third possible mechanism involves the stimulation of a pre-existing quiescent self-reactive B lymphocyte population.

In the first category evasion may occur in two possible ways: (1) because a particular body antigen is not accessible to the cells of the

Table 9.1 Mechanisms of autoantibody formation

1. **Evasion** of normal tolerance to 'self' antigens
   a. Hidden antigens
   b. Altered antigens —
      chemicals, drugs,
      infectious agents
2. **Breakdown** of tolerance mechanism
   a. Agents affecting antibody forming cells —
      chemicals, drugs,
      infectious agents
   b. Genetically determined lack of efficiency of tolerance control
      mechanisms (e.g. by suppressor T cells)
3. **Stimulation** of pre-existing B cell population capable of self-reactivity
   a. Infectious agents and adjuvants (? effects on suppressor T cells)

immune system as the antigen is hidden within a cell or tissue — these antigens are known as **sequestered** antigens; (2) because a tissue antigen is **altered** in some way by a chemical agent, a drug or an infectious agent.

Sequestered antigens. Hidden or sequestered antigens do seem to exist and the best examples of these are sperm antigens and lens antigen of the eye. Sperm can be shown to acquire an antigen during maturation which is absent from the immature germinal cells. Antibodies can be induced in the guinea-pig by immunising with autologous sperm showing that the immune system fails to recognise the sperm as part of self. Orchitis can be induced by combining the sperm with an adjuvant which gives a boost to the immune response, and at the same time in some way allows the stimulated lymphoid cells and antibody to gain access to the sperm-forming tissues. Orchitis in man is a rare complication of mumps infection in which it is assumed that the virus damages the basement membrane barrier of the seminiferous tubules and the cells of the immune system are thus allowed entry and initiate an immune response.

In the case of the lens it can be shown that if a rabbit is injected with bovine lens material, it develops antibodies which react with its own lens in vitro. Occasionally the surgical extraction of a lens for cataract is succeeded by inflammatory changes in retained lens substance sometimes affecting the other unoperated lens, and the same phenomenon can be induced experimentally in animals.

Interpretation of observations of this type is fraught with complications and can be regarded at present only as speculative evidence to support the concept of sequestered antigens as an initiating factor in autoimmune disease.

Altered antigens. Evidence in support of the second way in which normal tolerance mechanisms are circumvented is more concrete. Experimental studies of tolerance evasion by altered antigens have been carried out with purified proteins, conjugates of hapten and protein, and with cellular antigens. Some of the most definitive work is that carried out in America by Weigle who showed that rabbits made tolerant to bovine serum albumen (BSA) and then immunised with the cross-reacting antigen human serum albumen (HSA) eventually made antibodies which could react with BSA. The same result was obtained with chemically modified BSA. A closer approximation to autoimmune disease is provided by experiments using thyroglobulin in rabbits; not only are anti-rabbit thyroglobulin antibodies induced by injection of altered thyroglobulin but inflammatory lesions are also found in their thyroid glands.

Shared antigens. There has been considerable interest in the last few years in the role of microorganisms as a source of cross-reacting antigens sharing antigenic determinants with tissue components. The ability of viruses to bring about alterations of cell membranes has been suggested by studies on the effect of herpes and rabies viruses on tissue culture cells. New cell surface antigens (neoantigens), which appear to act as transplantation antigens, have been found in mouse cells infected with herpes and also with polyoma viruses.

There is an antigen in human colon extractable even from sterile fetal human colon, which is similar to a polysaccharide antigen present in *E. coli* 014. It is conceivable that the inflammatory condition of the colon known as ulcerative colitis, in which anti-colon antibodies are found, is due to an immune reaction initiated by the cross-reacting bacterial antigen. Similarly the Group A streptococci, which are closely associated with rheumatic fever, have an antigen in common with a human heart antigen. Heart lesions are a common finding in rheumatic fever and anti-heart antibody is found in just over 50% of patients with the condition.

Nephritogenic strains of Type 12 Group A streptococci carry surface antigens similar to those found in human glomeruli and infection by these organisms has been associated with the development of acute nephritis.

Drugs as haptens. Drugs can act as haptens (p. 194) which bind to tissue proteins. The resulting complex may be antigenic and result in an immune reaction which damages cells coated with the drug. An example of this is a metabolic breakdown product of the drug α-methyldopa (used in the treatment of hypertension). The immune response generated by these drug-altered cells can then result in haemolysis of the affected cells and α-methyldopa is thought to have the effect of altering or exposing normally hidden red cell antigens. The antibody which results has been found to combine with Rhesus antigens present on the surface of the patient's own normal erythrocytes. One hypothesis is that the α-methyldopa is incorporated into the Rhesus antigen when the red cell is being made and the change this induces prevents the antigen being recognised as self. (See also discussion of the effects of the drug Sedormid, p. 188).

Disturbed immunological mechanisms. The second main category of mechanisms by means of which autoimmune reactions may develop (Table 9.1) are those due to alteration in the cellular processes on which maintenance of normal tolerance depends. One way in which this might occur is by the direct effect of a chemical, a drug or an infectious agent on the lymphoid tissues. Alternatively, it is conceivable that the loss of normal tolerance control might be due to an inherited defect or lack of efficiency in the lymphoid cell population. The existence of a T lymphocyte population (suppressor T cells) that controls B lymphocyte activity has been noted on page 78. Suppressor T cells may prevent development of autoimmunity in the normal animal by recognising any idiotypic determinants (p. 69) of anti-self immunoglobulins expressed on the B cell surface. It is conceivable that a defect (inherited or induced) of such suppressor T cells might allow B cells of this type to escape and produce anti-self immunoglobulin.

There is much speculation amongst immunologists and clinicians on the role of infectious agents acting **directly** on the lymphoid tissues as a cause of autoimmune disease. This stems from the experimental evidence on the induction of autoimmune disease using tissue antigens combined with Freund's complete adjuvant. This water-in-oil emulsion owes its powerful stimulating effect on the lymphoid tissues, to killed mycobacteria which are incorporated in the oil. Without the mycobacterial component, tissue antigens are much less effective in disturbing the tolerance mechanisms. Rabbits injected with *Mycobacterium tuberculosis* alone have been shown to develop autoantibodies against a wide range of autologous tissues. The same phenomenon is found in a number of chronic infections in the human such as syphilis, actinomycosis and chronic tuberculosis. Infection with *Mycoplasma pneumoniae*, responsible for a disease known as primary atypical pneumonia, is associated with the development of IgM agglutinins in the patient's serum, which in the cold will react with the patient's own red cells.

A leukaemia virus has in the last few years been found in a strain of mice (New Zealand Black or NZB mice) characterised by the early development of autoimmune disease including autoimmune haemolytic anaemia and immune complex nephritis. The virus has been found in many body tissues and in the blood and can be seen in lymphoid organs, attached to the surface of lymphocytes. Similar virus particles have been found in embryos of the NZB strain, suggesting that it is passed through the placenta or is associated with the germ cells. The association of the virus with lymphocyte membranes has attracted the attention of immunologists and there has been speculation that the presence of the virus might interfere with normal lymphocyte reactivity to antigens. It is known (p. 78) that antigens can react with the lymphocyte surface and that this is probably one stimulus to immune transformation of these cells. The virus could conceivably upset the mechanisms controlling lymphocyte reactivity so that they respond abnormally to antigens to which they should remain tolerant. This idea receives some support from experiments in which animals stimulated with certain microorganisms (e.g. tubercle bacilli or corynebacteria) or the products of organisms (e.g. bacterial endotoxin) do not develop the expected immune tolerance when these antigens are administered in a way which would induce tolerance in the absence of the microbial product.

The human autoimmune disease systemic lupus erythematosus is characterised by anti-DNA antibodies and immune complexes containing DNA present in the kidneys (Fig. 9.8). Tubular structures resembling the nucleocapsids of myxo or paramyxoviruses have been found by electron microscopy in the endothelial cells of renal glomeruli and occasionally in the lymphocytes and joint tissues. Similar particles have been found in the tissues of patients with a number of other diseases in which autoantibodies are found (thyroiditis, myasthenia gravis, scleroderma and dermatomyositis). A

Fig. 9.8 Scheme showing pathogenic mechanisms in autoimmune disease with examples of disease states in each category

relationship between these findings and the pathogenesis of these diseases has not yet been established and is complicated by the difficulty in distinguishing between immune reactions directed against virus specified antigens and host antigens (autoantigens). Raised titres of antibody to various DNA and RNA viruses have been detected in patients with rheumatoid arthritis. Amongst these is the finding of an abnormally high incidence and titres of antibodies to the herpes virus, Epstein-Barr virus (EBV). Recent evidence suggests that there is a defect in the control by T lymphocytes of the expression of the virus by infected cells. Lymphocytes from RA patients, on exposure to EBV in vitro, transform more readily than do normal lymphocytes into EBV-containing lymphoblastoid cell lines secreting immunoglobulin. This immunoglobulin, if produced over a long period, would be likely to result in an antiimmunoglobulin response, some of which might be anti-idiotypic in nature (see p. 69). The anti-immunoglobulin rheumatoid factor could conceivably originate in this way.

Stimulation of pre-existing B cells. Another explanation for the development of auto-antibodies has recently been put forward (Table 9.1) — stimulation of a pre-existing population of lymphocytes (B cells) capable of making anti-self antibodies. In the mouse, cells making anti-red cell auto-antibodies can be induced to proliferate by the administration of substances with adjuvant activity (p. 62) e.g. certain corynebacteria and *B. pertussis.* Evidence indicating the presence of such lymphocytes was provided some years ago by a number of immunologists including the author, who described a variety of naturally occurring auto-antibodies in the serum of rodents. The availability of techniques such as immunocytoadherence and localised haemolysis in gel (p. 58) have now allowed the identification of the lymphocytes producing the auto-antibodies and thus put the earlier observations on a much firmer footing. It is a matter of speculation at present whether any human auto-immune state is a result of stimulation of these anti-self reactive lymphocytes. B lymphocytes capable of producing autoantibodies may increase in numbers with age. It is likely that in the normal individual proliferation of autoantibody producing B lymphocytes are held in check by immunoregulatory T lymphocytes.

There is little evidence that autoreactive T cells are present in the normal person. The possibility has been suggested that the autoreactive B cells are produced as a reaction to gut-derived antigens cross-reactive with self antigens. In a mouse model, autoantibody has been shown to first occur in lymph nodes draining the intestinal tract. If the mice were thymectomised neonatally, the autoantibodies did not appear, indicating the need for some T cell help. As indicated above, there is much evidence linking autoimmunity with exposure to a wide variety of infectious agents. It is possible that such agents can interfere with T cell regulation of autoreactive B lymphocytes without the direct participation of autoantigen in triggering the response.

Recent evidence suggests that B cells lose tolerance more readily than T cells and that T cells tolerant to self may be bypassed by presenting auto-antigens to B cells in a sufficiently immunogenic form perhaps combined with adjuvants as discussed above. If, as seems possible, the antibodies produced were of low affinity this would favour the development of toxic complexes with results as described on page 190.

HLA, immune response genes and disease susceptibility

The human lymphocyte antigen system (HLA system), consisting of several hundred genes on the short arm of chromosome 6, is described on page 162.

In Chapter 4 the important role performed by HLA-associated immune response genes is discussed in relation to the expression of acquired immunity. There has also been extensive search for associations between the expression of these genes and disease states.

In mice, some histocompatibility-associated Ir genes appear to predispose to autoimmune thyroiditis and susceptibility to viral meningitis infection. This suggests that these genes, possibly expressed as receptors on lymphocytes, may be important in genetic susceptibility or resistance to autoimmune diseases, infection and neoplasia.

The MHC locus can be thought of as a genetic locus which codes for cell surface structures important in various cell–cell interactions. Certain of the surface structures may provide selective advantages in providing protection against certain potentially dangerous disease states but, at the same time, may predispose to a limited number of somewhat rare diseases. In other words, such predisposition may be a minor inconvenience of a gene that confers a protective advantage (see also p. 131).

There are a number of different categories of association between the HLA complex and disease states. The first is a series of disease associations with different loci within the MHC, called the A, B, C and D loci. The best example is the association between ankylosing spondylitis and HLA-B27. However, the frequency of this locus in the population is about 8%, whilst the disease has a frequency of less than 0.1%. In those individuals who develop the disease and are not HLA-B27 there is a possible increase in HLA-A2 frequency. There is also a preponderance of males with the disease. A second category appears to be linked to the presence of two HLA-B loci, as in the case of juvenile-onset diabetes when there is an association with HLA-B8 and — BW15 loci. A third category is the incidence of, for example, sensitivity to ragweed allergen where a particular haplotype is inherited within a given family and appears to carry disease susceptibility. The implicated haplotype may vary from family to family, and the HLA identity only extends to siblings with the disease.

Table 9.2 shows that there are associations between specific HLA types and various chronic diseases, and that the association is much closer in some cases than in others. The fact that the association is not absolute may be due to the presence of other genes not linked to the HLA system. In support of this, multiple sclerosis has a much closer association (70% as against 15% of controls) with the MLC (mixed lymphocyte culture reaction) gene complex than with HLA types. Associations of diseases with individual HLA types imply that either increased resistance or susceptibility to the disease has been conferred by the HLA type. Positive associations suggest increased susceptibility, but an excess of a particular HLA type among the survivors of a disease with a high mortality suggests heightened resistance. One view explains the association by linking the Ir genes which are part of the MHC with the pathogenesis of those diseases in which an immune response is implicated. Another view is that HLA antigens or very closely linked gene products act as viral receptors or in other ways influence the pathogenesis of the condition. Environmental factors such as exposure to viruses may also be required for a susceptible individual to develop the disease, and the disease itself may have more than one aetiology.

Some recent work has provided further information on this difficult area that should make it possible to predict which women will develop autoimmune complications (SLE-like) if treated with Hydralazine, an antihypertensive drug. Women who are HLA DR4 positive and are slow acetylators always develop the autoimmune complication. Another development showing how a combination of apparently unrelated genetic markers can be used for accurate identification of a population at risk is the finding that a combination of HLA-B2/DR3 and a particular immunoglobulin allotype marker (p. 69) was associated with a 40-fold greater relative risk of developing chronic active hepatitis than if neither marker was pre-

Table 9.2 Some examples of disease association with HLA types

Disease	HLA type	Relative risk*
Ankylosing spondylitis		81
Reiter's syndrome	B27	48
Anterior uveitis		16.9
Juvenile arthritis		5
Coeliac disease		9.5
Addison's disease		3.9
Chronic active hepatitis	B8	2.9
Insulin-dependent diabetes		2.3
Thyrotoxicosis		2.3
Multiple sclerosis	B7	1.5
	DW2	5.0
Rheumatoid arthritis	DW4	
	DRW4	6.0
Ragweed allergy		
Early onset type 1 diabetes	HLA identity in siblings	

* Increased chance of having disease if individual is of particular HLA type

sent. Relapses in Graves' disease of the thyroid, associated with B27 can be accurately predicted by a combined analysis of HLA-DR3 status and Gm allotype. It therefore seems that investigation of genes for HLA antigen and immunoglobulin genes may lead to some useful information on susceptibility to disease.

There is little doubt that as further knowledge is gained of the HLA system, especially of the associated immune response genes (p. 98) and their role in the immune response itself, more insight will be gained into resistance or susceptibility to a variety of neoplastic, autoimmune and infectious diseases of man.

The pathogenesis of autoimmune disease
There is even more uncertainty in this area than exists with respect to the underlying abnormalities and stimuli which induce the autoimmune response.

Autoimmune diseases can be classified as **hypersensitivity** reactions on the basis of the definitions given in Chapter 6. These immune reactions, in contrast to those involved in protection from infectious disease, actually bring about severe and sometimes fatal reactions affecting the individual's own tissues and cells. The hypersensitivity reactions are divided into four types and three of these encompass autoimmune reactions.

Cytolytic or cytotoxic (type 2) reactions
The foremost of the autoimmune conditions in this category is autoimmune haemolytic anaemia. Here the antibodies are of two

main types: (1) antibodies of the IgM class which agglutinate the patient's own red cells in the cold; (2) antibodies of the IgG class which do not usually bring about direct agglutination of the red cells but can be detected by the Coombs test (p. 231) using an antiglobulin serum.

The anaemia is caused largely by the removal of antibody-coated cells in the spleen or the liver. Only rarely does lysis or agglutination take place to any extent in the circulation and involve the uptake of serum complement. Whilst normal red cells survive with a half-life in the circulation of just over three weeks, in this form of anaemia they are unlikely to have a half-life of more than one week.

Other forms of haemolytic anaemia exist including drug-induced types and those involving infective agents such as mycoplasma. Drugs involved include penicillin, phenacetin, quinine and α-methyldopa. The anaemia is brought about by the reaction of antibody with the drug linked as a hapten to the red cell surface, resulting in haemolysis. The precise details of the haptenic groups responsible for antigenic stimulation and their linkage to the red cell surface are uncertain. In mycoplasma infections the IgM cold agglutinins react with a widely distributed red cell antigen known as the I antigen.

Drug-induced agranulocytosis and thrombocytopoenia have also been described in which the leucocytes or platelets are destroyed by antibody directed at a complex of the drug and cell surface structures. Sedormid purpura has already been mentioned (p. 188).

Toxic-complex (type 3) reactions
Complexes of antibody and tissues antigens, particularly nuclear antigens (Fig. 9.8) are the cause of glomerulonephritis in a number of autoimmune states, notably in systemic lupus erythematosus where a wide range of anti-tissue antibodies is found, and in the similar type of disease of NZB mice. Complexes of antinuclear antibody and nuclear antigen, together with complement, can readily be demonstrated in the glomerular capillaries. The glomerular basement membranes become thickened and secondary changes develop in the renal tubules with progressive renal failure. The role of toxic complexes has been extensively studied in mice infected with lymphodytic chorio-meningitis virus (see p. 127). Some strains of mice develop toxic complex nephritis whilst others do not. Current evidence suggests that toxic-complex reactions are most likely to occur in strains of mice that produce low affinity antibodies and thus fail to eliminate antigen effectively. Clearance of immune complexes has been shown in rabbits and monkeys to be related to the number of antigen and antibody molecules in the complex. In

strains of mice prone to develop toxic-complex nephritis low affinity antibodies are produced and thus the complexes would have poor lattice structure (p. 223) and not be cleared from the circulation by phagocytic cells as effectively as larger aggregates.

Cell-mediated (type 4) reactions

There is no doubt that in both man and experimental animals the development of a number of autoimmune states is paralleled by the finding of cell-mediated reactions of the delayed hypersensitivity type as demonstrated by skin tests using tissue antigens. Whether the diseases are actually caused by immune reactions mediated by lymphoid cells is a matter of conjecture. Support for the role of cells in the disease process comes from studies in an experimental autoimmune disease known as autoimmune allergic encephalomyelitis. This is brought about by immunisation of animals with brain homogenate in Freund's complete adjuvant and paralysis follows demyelination of motor nerve fibres. The disease can be transferred in inbred strains of rats by the injection of lymphoid cells from affected animals to normal animals. The same type of transfer has been performed in autoimmune thyroiditis. In the latter condition it is proposed that the sensitised lymphocytes produce a surface injury to the cells of the thyroid acini and this allows the cytotoxic antibody, frequently present in the serum of affected subjects, to enter the cell and react with intracellular antigens.

That there may be an interaction between cell-mediated immunity and a humoral antibody is emphasised by work on autoimmune orchitis in guinea-pigs. Animals injected with a purified testis homogenate in Freund's complete adjuvant develop cell-mediated immunity (as shown by the development of delayed hypersensitivity on skin testing) but no circulating antibody or testicular lesion. When these animals are injected with anti-testis antibody (from a guinea-pig injected with testis homogenate in incomplete Freund's adjuvant, i.e. without tubercle bacilli) orchitis can be shown to develop. This interpretation is supported by the finding that anti-testis antibody enters the seminiferous tubules (as shown by the indirect fluorescent antibody method, p. 233) at the same time as cell-mediated immunity first appears (Fig. 9.8). Antibody-dependent cell-mediated cytotoxicity is described on page 189. The possibility that this form of reaction occurs in autoimmune states is supported by in vitro experimental work, but its role in vivo remains to be established.

Other diseases associated with autoimmune states

There is a large reservoir of diseases in which some form of autoantibody has been found but where neither the stimulus for auto-antibody formation nor the role, if any, of immune reactions has been elucidated.

Among these conditions is rheumatoid arthritis in which an IgM antibody called rheumatoid factor is present in the serum. This antibody is detected in vitro by its ability to agglutinate red cells or latex particles which have been coated with IgG globulin (p. 243). The rheumatoid factor does not appear to be directly involved in the pathogenesis of the disease and no satisfactory explanation has been offered to account for its pathogenesis. The possibility has been suggested that infective agents are involved, such as mycoplasma or chronic infective bacterial agents, and there are reports of the isolation of such agents from rheumatoid joints in man and in arthritis in a number of other species. One suggestion is that the infective agent may modify the lymphoid tissues so that there is a failure of the normal tolerance control mechanisms. Experimental arthritis can be induced in rats by the injection of Freund's complete adjuvant containing killed tubercle bacilli. This is a polyarthritis with mononuclear cell infiltration similar to the arthritis found in a human illness known as Reiter's syndrome, the main features of which are urethritis and arthritis and which may occur in the presence of a mycoplasma infection.

Recent evidence suggests that there may be an IgG form of rheumatoid factor present in both the blood and joint fluid of rheumatoid patients as well as the IgM type and that injection of autologous purified IgG into previously unaffected joints can induce actue arthritis. Further evidence suggesting that an antigen-antibody reaction is taking place is provided by the low complement levels found in patients' joint fluid and the presence of immune complexes.

Rheumatoid factors react with the Fc fragment of IgG (rabbit or human) but not with the Fab fragment. Rheumatoid factors are sometimes found in patients with diseases other than rheumatoid arthritis. These include systemic lupus erythematosus, Sjögren's syndrome, scleroderma, lymphoproliferative disease and in certain persistent bacterial, protozoal and viral infections. Even healthy subjects sometimes have low titres of the factor in their serum, particularly in the older age groups.

The mechanism underlying the appearance of these rheumatoid (anti-globulin) factors is not clear. In chronic infections it is conceivable that the factor is a response to antigenic determinants on the IgG molecule that are exposed when IgG antibody complexes with the infective agent. In the healthy individual a low titre of rheumatoid factor may perhaps serve a physiological function as a way of clearing degraded immunoglobulin molecules arising during infective or inflammatory processes. HLA-B27 individuals who become infected with salmonella, yersinia, shigella and gonococci often develop arthritis, suggesting that HLA-B27 acts in conjunction with the bacterial infection to cause the development of auto-antibodies.

Diabetes mellitus of the insulin-dependent type is believed to involve both an inherited susceptibility and environmental factors in the pathogenesis. The details of these interacting factors and their role are poorly understood. Susceptibility to the disease shows linkage to HLA haplotype inheritance within families, whatever the actual HLA phenotypes may be. A child that is of identical HLA phenotype to a diabetic sibling is likely to be susceptible. Autoantibody against pancreatic islet cells is found in these individuals, and when it is of the complement-fixing type seems to lead to islet cell damage. The antibody appears early in the disease before clinically obvious diabetes and serves as a marker of islet cell damage before progression to insulin insufficiency. This suggests the possibility for development of measures to arrest islet cell destruction before diabetes occurs.

Table 9.3 gives some examples of autoimmune diseases and the autoantibodies found.

Table 9.3 Examples of autoantibodies in disease

Disease	Autoantibody specificity
Autoimmune haemolytic anaemia	erythrocytes
Thrombocytopenic purpura	platelets
Systemic lupus erythematosus	nuclear antigens and antigens of various tissues and blood cells
Rheumatoid arthritis	immunoglobulin G
Primary biliary cirrhosis	mitochondria
Ulcerative colitis	colon lipopolysaccharide
Hashimoto's thyroiditis	thyroglobulin
Thyrotoxicosis	cell surface thyroid stimulating hormone (TSH) receptors
Pernicious anaemia	intrinsic factor
Myasthenia gravis	acetylcholine receptors (and certain muscle tissue)
Juvenile diabetes (type 1)	islet cell surface

Antibodies as a consequence of tissue damage

In considering the role of autoantibodies as a possible cause of autoimmune disease it should be remembered that antibodies of IgM type, directed at subcellular antigens, can be readily induced by various forms of tissue damage. These arise secondarily to the damage and appear to have no role in perpetuating it. Antibodies of this type have been shown in the author's laboratory and can readily be induced in rats by the injection of the hepatotoxic agent carbon tetrachloride. It was subsequently found that normal rats, mice and hamsters have some IgM anti-tissue antibody in their serum. A possible physiological role for these antibodies is suggested by the finding in vitro of a chemotactic effect on rat polymorphs of a mixture of the antitissue antibody and its antigen. Thus the antibody might be responsible for initiating a phagocytic cell clearing process to deal with the breakdown products of normal cell turnover.

Recent evidence indicates that IgG antibody existing in the normal individual seems to be able to recognise glycoprotein determinants which appear on aged red blood cells. These determinants are exposed following the loss of sialic acid groups from the outside of the cells on ageing. Their exposure can be reproduced experimentally by treatment with neuraminidase. The IgG antibodies bind to the exposed glycoprotein and enable the attachment of the red cell to the Fc receptors (p. 19) on a macrophage. The aged red cell is then phagocytosed and destroyed by the lysosomal enzymes of the macrophage.

All autoantibodies are therefore not necessarily autoregressive, although the history of immunity and protection inculcates the idea of antibodies acting solely as aggressive agents.

FURTHER READING

Hypersensitivity states
Austen F J, Block K J 1972 Biochemistry of acute allergic reactions. Blackwell, Oxford
Brostoff J 1973 Atopic allergy. British Journal of Hospital Medicine 9: 29
Cream J J 1973 Immune complex diseases. British Journal of Hospital Medicine 9: 8
Cochrane C G, Koffler D 1973 Immune complex disease in experimental animals and man. Advances in Immunology 18: 185
Lachmann P J, Peters D K 1982 Clinical aspects of immunology, 4th edn. Blackwell, Oxford
Turk J L 1967a Delayed hypersensitivity. In: Neuberger A, Tatum E L (eds) Frontiers in biology. North Holland, Amsterdam, vol 4
Turk J L 1967b Delayed hypersensitivity — specific cell-mediated immunity. British Medical Bulletin 23(1)
Turk J L 1969 Immunology in clinical medicine. Heinemann, London
Uhr J W 1966 Delayed hypersensitivity. Physiological Review 46: 359

Immune deficiency states
Ammann A J, Fudenberg H H 1976 In: Fudenberg H H, Stites D P, Caldwell J L, Wells J V (eds) Basic and clinical immunology. Lange, Los Altos
Asherson G L, Webster A D B 1980 Diagnosis and treatment of immunodeficiency diseases. Blackwell, Oxford

Lachmann P J, Peters D K 1982 Clinical aspects of immunology, 4th edn.
   Blackwell, Oxford
Martin N H 1970 The paraproteinaemias. British Journal of Hospital Medicine
   3: 662
Turk J L 1969 Immunology in clinical medicine. Heinemann, London
Waldenstrom J G 1968 Monoclonal and polyclonal hypergammaglobulinemia —
   clinical and biological significance. Cambridge University Press

Autoimmunity

Asherson G L 1968a The role of microorganisms in autoimmune responses. Progress
   in Allergy 12: 192
Asherson G L 1968a Autoantibody production as a breakdown of immune tolerance.
   In: Cinader B (ed) Regulation of the antibody response. Thomas, Springfield,
   Illinois, p 68
Burnet F M 1959 The clonal selection theory of acquired immunity. Cambridge
   University Press
Cudworth A G 1980 Current concepts in the aetiology of type 1 (insulin-dependent)
   diabetes mellitus. In: Bellingham A J (ed) Advanced medicine 16. Pitman,
   London, p 123
Freedman S O, Gold P 1979 Clinical immunology, 2nd edn. Harper and Row,
   London
Holborow E J (ed) 1981 Clinics in immunology and allergy. Autoimmunity.
   W B Saunders, Philadelphia
Irvine W J (ed) 1979 Medical immunology. Teviot Scientific Publications,
   Edinburgh
Lachmann P J, Peters D K (eds) 1982 Clinical aspects of immunology. Blackwell,
   Oxford
Levy J A 1974 Autoimmunity and neoplasia: the possible role of C-type viruses.
   American Journal of Clinical Pathology 62: 258
McDevitt H C, Bodmer F 1974 HL-A, immune response genes and disease. Lancet
   1: 1269
Marmion B P 1976 A microbiologist's view of investigative rheumatology. In:
   Dumonde D C (ed) Infection and immunology in the rheumatic diseases.
   Blackwell, Oxford, p 245
Marmion B P, MacKay J M K 1977 Rheumatoid arthritis and the viral hypothesis.
   Bayer symposium VI: Experimental models of chronic inflammatory diseases.
   Springer-Verlag, Berlin, p 188
Moller G 1975 HLA and disease. Transplant Review 22: 2
Samter M 1965 Immunologic diseases. Little Brown, Boston
Talal N, Fyek M 1976 Autoimmunity. In: Fudenberg H H, Stites D P, Caldwell
   J L, Wells J V (eds) Basic and clinical immunology. Lange, Los Altos
Trentin J J 1967 Cross-reacting antigens and neo-antigens (with implications for
   autoimmunity and cancer immunity). Williams and Wilkins, Baltimore
Turk J L 1969 Immunology in clinical medicine. Heinemann, London
Weir D M, Elson C J 1969 Anti-tissue antibodies and immunological tolerance to
   self. Arthritis and Rheumatism 12: 254
Willoughby D A, Giroud J P (eds) 1980 Inflammation mechanisms and treatment.
   MTP Press, London
World Health Organisation 1977 Immune complexes in disease. Report of a WHO
   scientific group. WHO, Technical report series no. 606

10

Interaction of antibody with antigen and applications in laboratory investigations

Objectives

On completion of this section the reader will be able to:

1. Describe the difference between the primary interaction of antigen and antibody and the secondary effects of this union
2. With the aid of a diagram, describe a precipitation reaction in terms of optimal proportions
3. Give two examples of immunodiffusion in gels
4. Describe agglutination and give three examples of practical applications
5. Outline the stages in a complement fixation test
6. Describe an antiglobulin test and explain how the same principle is used in the fluorescent antibody techniques and the ELISA test
7. Describe the principle of radioimmunoassay
8. Give four examples of the use of antibody-antigen reactions in the clinical laboratory
9. Describe, with examples, the investigation of immune deficiency states
10. Give two methods for the detection of immune complexes.

An antibody, as has been pointed out, is an immunoglobulin molecule secreted into the tissue fluids from lymphoid cells which have been exposed to a foreign substance — an antigen. An antigen may be potentially harmful, such as bacterium or virus, or it may be a harmless bland substance such as foreign serum protein. The antibody can combine only with antigen which is identical or nearly identical with the inducing antigen and not with unrelated antigens. When molecules of antibody and antigen are brought together in solution, they interact with each other by the formation of a link between an antigen-binding site on the immunoglobulin molecule — part of the Fab fragment — and the particular chemical groupings which make up what is termed the antigenic determinant of the antigen molecule. The molecules are held together by **non-**

covalent intermolecular forces which are effective only when the antigen-binding site and the antigenic determinant group are able to make close contact. The better the fit, the closer the contact and the stronger the antigen-antibody bond. These factors determine what is often called the **affinity** of the antibody molecule. Antibodies of varying combining quality exist and the overall tendency to combine with antigen is the average ability of the antibodies to combine with antigen or the average intrinsic association constant. This can be calculated experimentally by application of the concepts of chemical equilibria to antigen-antibody interactions. Studies of this type have shown that the affinity of antibodies increases as immunisation proceeds and that the dose of antigen can influence the quality of antibody (see p. 88).

The methods used for the detection of antigen-antibody reactions in the laboratory fall in two functional groups: first, procedures designed to elucidate the cytodynamics of antibody formation which involve the study of the behaviour of single cells or small populations of cells; the second group, which is the subject of the present discussion, concerns the detection and quantitation of **secreted antibody** circulating in the blood or present in the tissue fluids.

The methods used here range in their application from highly specialised studies of the physico-chemical aspects of antigen-antibody interaction to widely used procedures designed to aid in the diagnosis of disease.

Primary interaction and secondary effects
In practical terms, the union of antibody with antigen can be detected at two different levels. The first level is that following **primary union** of the two reactants and usually requires that one or other reactant is labelled with a suitable marker such as a fluorescent dye or a radioactive isotope. A simple example of this is the microscopic localisation in a tissue of a particular microorganism utilising an antiserum prepared against the microorganism and labelled with a dye that fluoresces under UV light. A widely used method in experimental immunology makes use of the fact that immunoglobulins are insoluble in 50% saturated ammonium sulphate. The test developed by Farr uses antigen labelled with ^{131}I that is mixed with antibody-containing serum and left to equilibrate. Ammonium sulphate solution is then added to the mixture resulting in the precipitation of the antibody together with any labelled antigen bound to it. The unbound antigen remains in solution (only

antigens that are themselves soluble in 50% ammonium sulphate can be used in this form of the test). The quantity of isotope-labelled antigen bound to the salt-precipitated antibody is then estimated by placing the washed precipitate in radioactive counting equipment. This sensitive and useful technique is a measure of the capacity of an antiserum to bind antigen.

The second level at which antigen-antibody combination can be detected depends on the development, after primary union, of certain changes in the physical state of the complex, resulting in precipitation or agglutination of the components or, alternatively, in the activation of non-antibody components such as serum complement or histamine from mast cells. Reactions of this type occurring subsequent to primary union are termed **secondary phenomena**. This discussion is concerned with the principles of a few of these secondary phenomena which are in common use.

Secondary effects; interpretation and applications. Before considering these reactions individually, it is important to be aware of the difficulties in interpreting results of such tests. The initiation and development of the secondary phenomena constitute a complicated series of events involving many variables such as the type of antibody taking part, the relative proportions of antibody and antigen, characteristics of the antigen molecule, presence of electrolytes, inhibitory substances and unstable components.

Despite these formidable difficulties, the widely and long-used secondary phenomena such as precipitation, agglutination and complement fixation have an important role to play as aids in the diagnosis of disease and in the identification of microorganisms.

The secondary phenomena can bring about several readily observable changes when carried out in vitro. These are used in tests to demonstrate the presence of antibody in the sera of patients suffering from infectious disease, or producing an antibody response to cell antigens as might, for example, occur after incompatible blood transfusion, tissue grafting or in autoimmune states.

Reactions of this type can also be used to identify antigens in the tissues or body fluids and, for example, would be utilised for blood grouping, tissue typing or the identification of microorganisms.

Among the most important of these reactions are **precipitation**, which occurs between antibody and antigen molecules in soluble form; **agglutination**, in which the antibodies directed against surface antigens of particulate materials such as microorganisms or erythrocytes, link them together in large clumps or aggregates; and

complement fixation in which antibody molecules, after reaction with antigen, activate the complex blood components that make up serum complement.

In addition to these widely used serological tests, a number of other effects of antigen-antibody interaction are of medical importance. These include **neutralisation** tests used for example in virus identification, **immobilisation** tests with bacteria and protozoa and **skin tests** for the reaginic antibody characteristic of anaphylactic states.

Precipitation

Optimal proportions. As a result of the interaction of antibody and antigen molecules in solution, complexes of the two types of molecule will form and precipitation may occur depending on the relative concentration of the two reactants. If a series of tubes is set up (Fig. 10.1), each containing a constant amount of antiserum, and decreasing amounts of antigen are added to the tubes in the row, a haziness will start to appear in the tubes gradually increasing to clearly visible **aggregates** or **precipitates**. The amount of precipitation will be seen to increase along the row, reaching a maximum and then falling off with the lower antigen concentration. The tubes where most precipitate appears contain the **optimal proportions** of antigen and antibody for precipitation. The composition of the precipitate varies with the original proportions of the antibody and antigen; if antigen is in excess the precipitate will contain relatively more of this component and similarly more antibody if it is present

| Antigen | Neat | $\frac{1}{2}$ | $\frac{1}{4}$ | $\frac{1}{8}$ | $\frac{1}{16}$ | $\frac{1}{32}$ |

Antibody   Neat in each tube

Fig. 10.1

in excess. As can be seen from Figure 10.2, on the antigen excess side of optimal proportions less precipitate appears. This is due to the inability of the antigen-antibody complexes formed to link up to other complexes and so make a large aggregate or lattice which will appear as a visible precipitate (tube 1, Fig. 10.2). Large aggregates of antibody and antigen can form best under conditions of optimal proportions where the antibody and antigen proportions are such that after initial combination of the molecules, free antigen-binding sites and antigen determinant groups remain, enabling the complexes to link up into a large lattice formation (as in tube 2 of Fig. 10.2). In antibody excess all the free determinants of the antigen molecule are soon taken up with antibody, so that very little linking can take place between the complexes (as in tube 3 of Fig. 10.2).

Applications. The precipitin test can be carried out in a quantitative manner by estimating the protein content of the precipitate at optimal proportions. The qualitative test is much more widely used and is of considerable value in detecting and identifying antigens, having applications in the typing of streptococci or pneumococci. This is done by layering an extract of the organism over antiserum. After a short while, a ring of precipitate forms at the interface (this is called the ring test). The technique is also used in forensic stud-

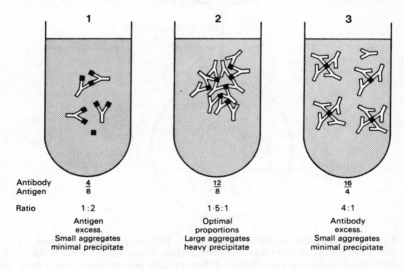

	1	2	3
Antibody	4	12	16
Antigen	8	8	4
Ratio	1:2	1·5:1	4:1
	Antigen excess. Small aggregates minimal precipitate	Optimal proportions Large aggregates heavy precipitate	Antibody excess. Small aggregates minimal precipitate

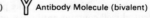

■ Antigen Molecule (can react with 4 antibody molecules)   Ⴞ Antibody Molecule (bivalent)

Fig. 10.2

ies and in detecting adulteration of foodstuffs. A modification of the test in which precipitation is allowed to occur in **agar gel** is very widely used for detecting the presence of antibody in serum or antigen in unknown preparations, and is valuable for showing the identity of different antigen preparations (Fig. 10.3). A concentration gradient forms in the gel, the concentration of a substance decreasing as the molecules diffuse away from the well in which they were placed. **Precipitin bands** form in the gel in the position where the antigen and antibody molecules reach optimal proportions after diffusion.

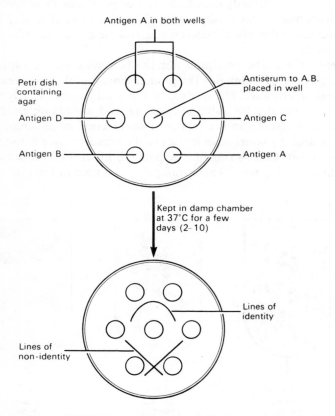

Fig. 10.3 Immunodiffusion or gel diffusion test. Wells are cut in a layer of agar in a Petri dish. Antiserum and antigen solutions are placed opposite each other in the wells and after allowing a few days for diffusion to take place precipitin bands will form where antibody and antigen meet in suitable proportions (optimal proportions). No reactions take place with antigens C and D as the antiserum in the central well contains antibodies only for antigens A and B. Lines of identity as formed between the two A wells enable the technique to be used for identifying unknown antigens

When a large number of different antigens are present in a solution, it is difficult to separate the precipitin bands for each of the antigen-antibody reactions by the simple gel-diffusion method just described. In such a situation, a variation of this method can be used to identify the individual components. This modification is particularly valuable in analysing a multicomponent system such as serum. The individual components of serum are first separated by electrophoresis in agar gel and an antiserum, prepared against the serum, is allowed to diffuse towards the separated components, resulting in the formation of precipitin bands (Fig. 10.4). This

Fig. 10.4 Immunoelectrophoresis. The antigen, for example, serum, is placed in a small well cut in a layer of agar on a microscope slide. A direct current is applied and differential migration of the serum components takes place. (They are not normally visible in the agar and will show up only if suitably stained.) After electrophoresis for an hour or so, a trough is cut longitudinally in the agar and an antiserum against the electrophoresed antigen is placed in the trough. The two components diffuse towards each other and precipitin bands form. These can be shown up more clearly by staining with a protein stain. This is a very powerful analytic technique and can show up about 30 different components in human serum compared with 4 or 5 by electrophoresis

method, known as **immunoelectrophoresis**, is particularly valuable for showing the presence of abnormal globulin constituents in the serum of patients with myelomatosis and other serum protein abnormalities.

A microimmunodiffusion test with wells cut in a layer of agar on a microscope slide is a convenient modification of the Petri dish method. This procedure has been used for the detection in human serum of the **Hepatitis B antigen** which is associated with serum hepatitis. The routine screening of blood products by this technique using specific antisera prepared in animals is likely to become an important laboratory test in the prevention of serum hepatitis outbreaks (see also p. 236).

Instead of placing antibody and antigen in separate wells and allowing them to diffuse towards each other, the antibody can be incorporated in the agar and the antigen placed in wells. This technique is known as **single radial immunodiffusion** and depends upon diffusion of antigen from the well until a point is reached where the concentration is optimal for precipitation to occur. Close to the antigen well the concentration of antigen will be high and although the antigen will combine with antibody in the agar, the complexes will be unable to form the large lattice structure necessary for precipitation to take place (Fig. 10.2) and will thus remain as soluble complexes. The precipitin band that forms at optimal proportions of antigen and antibody will show up as a ring around the antigen well. The distance the ring forms from the antigen well will be dependent on the concentration of the antigen in the well. In practice the **diameter** of the ring is measured around a well containing an unknown concentration of antigen and this is compared with the diameter of the rings formed with known concentrations of the antigen, thus enabling the estimation of the concentration of antigen in the unknown preparation.

This technique is widely used to estimate the quantity of the various immunoglobulin classes in human serum samples. An antiserum to a particular immunoglobulin class (e.g. IgG) is incorporated in the agar and the test serum sample is placed in a well. The diameter of the precipitation band that forms after incubation is then compared to the diameter obtained with standard IgG prepparations of known concentration. The diameters of the rings with the **standard** IgG preparations (e.g. 3 or 4 dilutions of a known concentration) can be plotted graphically against the concentration of IgG and the diameter obtained with the unknown sample can be read of against concentration on this reference graph (Fig. 10.5)

Fig. 10.5 Diagram of single radial immunodiffusion plate with antiserum incorporated in agar and antigen dilutions and test sample in wells. Reference graph drawn using 3 concentrations of antigen standard showing the diameter of precipitin ring obtained with each concentration (●). Diameter of unknown sample (○) when plotted enables determination of its antigen concentration

Agglutination

In this reaction the antigen is part of the surface of some particulate material such as a red cell, bacterium or perhaps an inorganic particle (e.g. polystyrene latex) which has been coated with antigen. Antibody added to a suspension of such particles combines with the surface antigens and links them together to form clearly-visible aggregates or **agglutinates** (Fig. 10.6). In its simplest form an agglutination test is set up in round-bottomed test tubes or perspex plates with round-bottomed wells and doubling dilutions of the antiserum are made up in the tubes (neat, 1:2, 1:4, 1:8, etc). The particulate antigen is then added and after incubation at 37°C agglutination is seen in the bottom of the tubes. The last tube showing clearly visible agglutination is the end point of the test. The reciprocal of the antiserum at the end point, e.g. 1/256, is known as the the **titre** of the antiserum and is a measure of the number of antibody units per unit volume of serum, e.g. if the end point occurs at a 1/256 dilution of the antiserum and if the test has been carried out in 1 ml volumes, the titre of the serum is 256 units per ml of serum.

One practical difficulty of importance in agglutination tests is the occasional inhibition of agglutination in the first tubes of an antiserum dilution series, agglutination occurring only in those tubes containing more dilute antiserum. This is known as the **prozone**

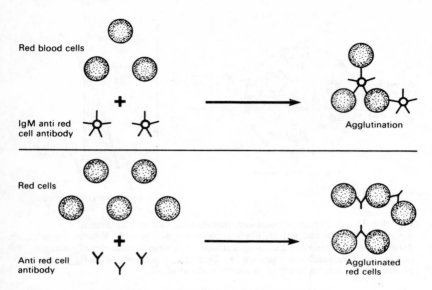

Fig. 10.6 Agglutination reaction. The IgM molecule, with at least five
antigen-binding sites, is particularly effective in bringing about agglutination

phenomenon and is probably, in part, due to the stabilising effects
of high protein concentration on the particles. The protein coats the
particles, increases their net charge and so brings about increased
electrostatic repulsion between individual particles, thus opposing
the efforts of the antibody molecules to link the particles together.
However, once the protein concentration is reduced by dilution the
antibody molecules can then exert their aggregating effect and
bring about agglutination. The agglutination reaction has been
shown to require the presence of electrolytes in the suspending
medium and is usually performed for this reason at physiological
salt concentration.

Applications. One of the classical applications of the agglutination test in diagnostic bacteriology is the **Widal test** used for the
demonstration of antibodies to salmonellae in serum specimens taken
from suspected enteric fever cases. Agglutination is the basic technique used in blood grouping, the A, B or O group of the red cells
under test being determined by agglutination with a specific antiserum — an anti-A serum for example will agglutinate A cells but
not B or O cells. Red cells and inert particles such as polystyrene
latex can be coated with various antigens and suitably coated
particles are used in a variety of diagnostic tests such as thyroid

Fig. 10.7 Principle of hormone assay by agglutination inhibition. Red cells coated with hormone are agglutinable by anti-hormone antibody. The addition to the antiserum of a test sample containing free hormone will block the antigen-binding sites and prevent agglutination. The test can be carried out quantitatively by comparing the activity of a known standard hormone preparation with the test sample

antibody tests using thyroglobulin-coated cells or latex particles. Hormone-coated red cells or inert particles are used in many hormone assay procedures which are based on the inhibition of the antibody-induced agglutination of the hormone-coated particles by hormone added in the sample under test (Fig. 10.7). Tests of this type are in wide use in pregnancy diagnosis.

Certain viruses, e.g. the myxoviruses causing influenza and mumps, have the property of bringing about agglutination of red cells (haemagglutination). **Inhibition of haemagglutination** by antibody in patients' serum is a widely-used diagnostic procedure. The presence of antibody in the patient's serum is thus detected by its ability to link with virus particles and prevent them from bringing about agglutination of the red cells (Fig. 10.8).

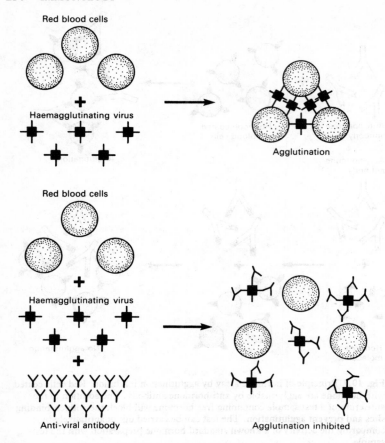

Fig. 10.8 Virus haemagglutination inhibition test. Red cell agglutination is brought about by a variety of viruses (see text). This can be inhibited by mixing the virus with anti-viral antibody as shown in the diagram. The test can be quantitated by comparison of serial dilutions of virus alone and virus-antibody mixture

IgM antibodies capable of agglutinating human red cells (including those of the individual producing the antibody) between 0 and 4°C are sometimes found in certain human diseases including primary atypical pneumonia, malaria, trypanosomiasis and acquired haemolytic anaemia.

The presence of antibody globulin on a red cell may not result in direct agglutination of the cells, for example in some Rh-negative mothers with Rh-positive infants or in acquired haemolytic anaemia. It is, however, possible to show that the red cells are coated with antibody by using an **antiglobulin** serum (produced in the rabbit by

Anti-red-cell antibody
combined with buried
surface antigen

Red cell
membrane

Antiglobulin

Antiglobulin combines with attached
anti-red-cell antibody and links cells
together for agglutination

Fig. 10.9 Coombs antiglobulin test. The red cell antibody, probably because it is directed against an antigen situated deep in the cell wall, cannot link two red cells together for agglutination. The addition of an antiglobulin serum brings about agglutination by linking two attached immunoglobulins to one another

injecting human globulin) which will bring about agglutination of the cells (Fig. 10.9). This is the basis of the Coombs test which is a very widely used serological procedure.

Complement fixation
The fact that antibody, once it combines with antigen, is able to activate the complement system is used as a way of showing the presence of a particular antibody in a serum, e.g. the **Wassermann** antibody in syphilis, or in identifying an antigen such as a virus.

The complement of most species will react with antibody derived from other species and guinea-pig serum is a common laboratory source of complement. Some of the components of complement are heat-labile and are destroyed by heating at 56°C for 20 to 30 minutes. The individual components of the complement system are taken up by the antigen-antibody complex in a particular order and destruction of the heat-labile components which are taken up early prevents the remaining components from taking part (see p. 21).

For most antigens the reaction of the complement system with the antigen-antibody complex causes in itself no visible effect, and it is necessary to use an indicator system consisting of sheep red cells coated with anti-sheep red cell antibody. Complement has the ability to lyse the antibody-coated cells, probably by virtue of the esterase activity of one of the components acting on the red cell membrane. In a test the antibody, complement and antigen are first mixed together and after a period of incubation the indicator system, antibody-coated sheep cells, are added. The complement will, however, have been taken up during the incubation stage by the original antibody-antigen complex and will not be available to lyse the red cells. Thus, a **positive** complement fixation test is indicated by **absence of lysis** of the red cells whilst a negative test, with unused complement, is shown by lysis of the red cells (Fig. 10.10).

Applications. The classical complement fixation test is the Wassermann reaction used in the diagnosis of syphilis. The test system consists of Wassermann antigen mixed with dilutions of the patient's serum in the presence of guinea-pig complement. After the antigen and patient's serum have had time to react and take up the limited amount of complement available in the system, the indicator system is added to show whether or not there is free complement. Controls are included to ensure that none of the reagents are anti-complementary (able to take up complement nonspecifically as might, for example, occur with contaminated serum) and positive and negative control sera are tested in parallel. Complement fixation tests are used routinely for detecting viruses in tissue cultures which have been inoculated with specimens of blood or tissue fluids from humans with probable virus infections.

INDICATOR SYSTEM

Complement | Sheep red cell coated with anti-sheep red cell antibody | Complement reacts with anti-sheep red cell antibody and lyses cell

POSITIVE TEST

Antigen | Antibody to antigen | Complement | Antibody reacts with antigen and complement combines | No lysis of antibody coated red cells as complement used up

Fig. 10.10 Complement-fixation test. The indicator system (sheep red cells coated with antibody to sheep red cells) is normally lysed in the presence of complement (fresh guinea-pig serum) — top. If another antibody-antigen system is first mixed with the complement it will no longer be available to lyse the indicator system — bottom

Antigen-antibody reactions using fluorescent labels

The precise localisation of tissue antigens or the antigens of infecting organisms in the body, of anti-tissue antibody and of antigen-antibody complexes was achieved by the introduction of the use of fluorochrome-labelled proteins by Coons and Kaplan in 1950. The adsorption of ultraviolet light between 290 and 495 nm by fluorescein and its emission of longer wavelength green light (525 nm) is used to visualise protein labelled with this dye. The technique is more sensitive than precipitation or complement fixation techniques, and fluorescent protein tracers can be detected at a concentration of the order of 1 μg protein per ml body fluid.

Applications. Some of the uses to which the technique has been put include the localisation of the origin of a variety of serum protein components, for example immunoglobulin production by plasma cells and other lymphoid cells. The demonstration and localisation in the tissues of antibody globulin in a variety of autoimmune conditions has been shown, including an anti-nuclear antibody in the serum of patients with systemic lupus erythematosus and thyroid auto-antibodies in the sera of patients with Hashimoto's thyroiditis. In the diagnostic field most human pathogens can be demonstrated by immunofluorescence and a tentative diagnosis may be made much sooner than by cultivation. The fluorescent method at present can be used to supplement rather then replace conventional methods.

There are two main procedures in use, the direct and indirect methods (Fig. 10.11). The **direct method** consists of bringing fluorescein-tagged antibodies into contact with antigens fixed on a slide (e.g. in the form of a tissue section or a smear of an organism), allowing them to react, washing off excess antibody and examining under the UV light microscope. The site of union of the labelled antibody with its antigen can be seen by the apple-green fluorescent areas on the slide. The **indirect method** can be used both for detecting specific antibodies in sera or other body fluids and also for identifying antigens. This method differs from the direct method in the use of a non-labelled antiserum which is layered on first, in the same way as described above. Whether or not this antiserum has reacted with the material on the slide is shown by means of a fluorescein-tagged **antiglobulin serum** specific for the globulin of the serum applied first. Such an antiglobulin serum can be used to detect antibody globulin in sera to a variety of different antigens which gives it a considerable advantage over the direct test; it is also more sensitive.

Other types of labelled antibody test have been developed on the same principles as the fluorescent methods. Horseradish peroxidase

234   IMMUNOLOGY

Fluorescein
tagged
antibody

Antigen

Attached fluorescein
tagged antibody
visualized by
U.V. microscopy

INDIRECT METHOD
First Step
Untagged
antibody

Antibody attached
to antigenic
determinant

Second Step

Fluorescein
tagged
antiglobulin

Attached fluorescein
tagged antiglobulin
visualized by
U.V. microscopy

Fig. 10.11 Fluorescent antibody technique — direct and indirect methods. The indirect method can be seen to be more sensitive as two or more fluorescein-tagged antiglobulin molecules can be attached to each immunoglobulin molecule bound to its antigen

can readily be linked to antibody leaving the antibody still able to combine with its antigen. After this has occurred (e.g. in a tissue section layered with the peroxidase-labelled antibody and then washed) the site of localisation of the antibody can be visualised by conventional histochemical staining of the peroxidase using its substrate (the peroxidase reaction). Ferritin (an electron-dense blood pigment) conjugated antibody has also been used in electron-microscope studies to show the localisation of cell antigens.

Cytotoxic tests
Tests of this type are used in combination with red blood cell agglutination for studying histocompatibility antigen systems in tissue typing.

The cytotoxic test consists essentially of determining whether or not the **permeability** of cells changes after their incubation with antibody and complement (Fig. 10.12). Cytotoxic antibody, after combination with the target cell, will activate complement components and bring about changes in permeability of the cell membrane. The permeability changes can affect the ability of the cell to exclude a dye such as trypan blue which will penetrate the cell and be visible by simple microscopic examination.

NEGATIVE TEST—No antibody

- Trypan blue dye
- Leucocyte
- Complement
- Dye excluded from cell

POSITIVE TEST—Antibody present

Complement reacts with antibody and makes cell membrane permeable to dye

Trypan blue enters cell

Antibody

Fig. 10.12 Cytotoxic test

Although the test is applicable to a wide range of nucleated cells and is the test of choice with blood leucocytes, it is rather less sensitive than the red cell haemagglutination tests and more laborious to perform.

Radioimmunoassay methods

Increasing use has been made over the last few years of immunologically based assay methods for the accurate quantitative estimation of **polypeptide hormones**. These methods offer a unique combination of specificity, precision and simplicity and are already available for the assay of some 14 of the 20 or so polypeptide hormones in man. Monoclonal antibodies are now used extensively in the tests.

The principle of the assay methods is that radio-iodine labelled (purified) hormone competes with the non-labelled hormone of a sample under test, for the anti-hormone antibody with which the labelled and non-labelled hormone are mixed. The more of the hormone in the test sample the less chance the labelled hormone has of combining with the limited number of antibody molecules that are available in the anti-hormone serum. Thus by measuring the quantity of labelled hormone combined with antibody (using isotope counting equipment) a measure of the hormone in the test sample can be obtained. The more labelled hormone combined with antibody, the lower the hormone level in the test sample. The quantity of isotope labelled hormone complexing with the anti-hormone antibody varies inversely with the quantity of unlabelled hormone in the test sample.

In order to measure the amount of labelled hormone attached to antibody it is necessary to separate the hormone-antibody complexes from the mixture. A variety of methods have been developed to achieve this, perhaps the most common being electrophoretic separation. Provided the **free** hormone has a different electrophoretic mobility from the antibody globulin then separation of hormone **bound** to antibody is straightforward. Other methods of separation depend upon the antibody being linked to an insoluble support (e.g. cellulose). The insoluble complex is then mixed with labelled and test hormone (tube 1, Fig. 10.13), allowed to interact (tube 2, Fig. 10.13) and later the unreacted hormone is removed and the amount of labelled hormone attached to the insoluble complex is measured (tube 3, Fig. 10.13).

An assay for IgE levels in serum has been developed using iodine labelled IgE and anti-IgE linked to cellulose, and assays using these principles are being developed for the detection of hepatitis B antigen in human serum.

Immunoassays using enzyme-linked antibody or antigen

Enzyme-linked immunosorbent assay (ELISA)

Labels other than radioactive isotopes and fluorescent dyes can be linked on to antibody or antigen molecules. There has been recent interest in the use of enzymes such as horseradish peroxidase or alkaline phosphatase linked to antibody or antigen molecules. The presence of the enzyme linked molecule is detected by means of the enzyme substrate and can be measured by spectrophotometry. Either the labelled antigen or the antibody can be attached to an insoluble support, such as plastic beads or plastic agglutination plates. After the material has attached and the excess has been washed away, enzyme-linked antigen or antibody is added, together with the test substance. The antigen or antibody (whichever is being measured) in the test solution competes with the added labelled antigen or antibody reagent for the material attached to the

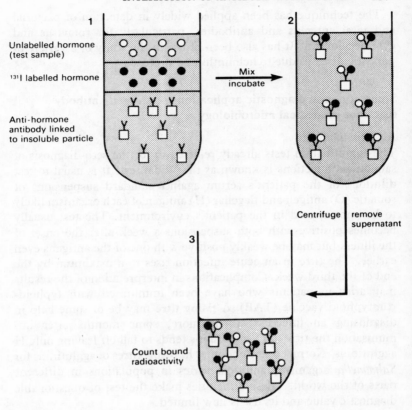

Fig. 10.13 Illustration of the use of antihormone antibody linked to an insoluble particle for the assay of the amount of hormone in a test sample. The quantity of ^{131}I labelled hormone complexing with the anti-hormone antibody varies inversely with the amount of unlabelled hormone in the test sample. A standard curve can be prepared using known concentrations of purified hormone in the same way as illustrated in Fig. 10.5. This will enable the result obtained with the test sample to be plotted and its concentration obtained

plastic plates. The amount of enzyme-labelled reagent can then be estimated by the addition of enzyme substrate. The product of the reaction between enzyme and substrate is finally determined by spectrophotometry.

There are a number of variations of the technique similar to those used with fluorescent antibodies. These include a sandwich technique with antigen bound to the plastic plate, the antibody to be assayed as the second layer and enzyme linked to immunoglobulin as the top layer. Enzyme substrate is finally added and the product determined by colour change in the spectrophotometer.

The technique has been applied widely in detection of bacterial and viral antigens and antibodies, particularly for rotavirus and cytomegalovirus. It has also been of use in the study of a variety of parasitic diseases due to helminths and protozoa.

Some common diagnostic applications of antigen-antibody reactions in medical microbiology

Agglutination tests

The agglutination tests already referred to for the sero-diagnosis of salmonella infections is known as the Widal test. It is usual to test dilutions of the patient's serum against standard suspensions of somatic (O) antigen and flagellar (H) antigen of each organism likely to be encountered in the patient's environment. The test usually becomes positive with both suspensions a week after the onset of the illness but may be weakly positive with one of the antigens even earlier. The titre in an acute infection rises to a maximum by the end of the third week. Complications in interpretation of the results may arise in patients who have been immunised with typhoid-paratyphoid vaccine (TAB). A **rising titre** may be of some help in diagnosing an infection; furthermore, some months after immunisation the titre of O agglutinins tends to fall off leaving only H agglutinins. Normal sera sometimes have low titres of agglutinins for *Salmonella* organisms and this varies in populations in different parts of the world. These difficulties make the test of questionable diagnostic value and its use is now limited.

Another widely used agglutination test is the **Paul-Bunnell** reaction. This is used for the diagnosis of infectious mononucleosis in which agglutinins develop for sheep erythrocytes. Normal serum may agglutinate sheep cells in low dilutions and a titre of 128 is taken as suggestive and 256 as positive for the test. In some individuals who have received horse serum as a therapeutic agent (e.g. anti-tetanus serum) agglutinins develop for sheep cells because of the presence in the horse serum of an antigen very widespread in nature, known as the **Forssman** antigen. This antigen is present in the red cells of sheep and the cells of a number of other species, including the guinea-pig. The usual way of differentiating the two types of antibody is to mix the serum with minced guinea-pig tissue (usually kidney). This treatment will absorb out the anti-Forssman antibody leaving the anti-sheep cell antibody unaffected. Ox red cells, which contain both the Forssman antigen and an antigen similar to that on sheep cells which reacts with the Paul-Bunnell antibody, will absorb out both types of antibody.

Complement fixation tests
These tests, described on page 231, have wide application in the diagnosis of bacterial and viral infections. One of the most commonly used methods is the Wassermann test used in the diagnosis of **syphilis**. This reaction depends upon the fixation of complement by the patient's antibody after it has reacted with cardiolipin, an alcoholic extract (a phosphatide lipoid) from normal animal tissues, usually ox heart. Why antibodies against this material develop in syphilis is not clear. Some workers suggest that it results from autoimmunisation with host lipids made antigenic in some way by the spirochaete (*Trep. pallidum*) responsible for syphilis, whilst others believe that the spirochaete contains a cell wall antigen related to the tissue antigen (p. 28).

Interpretation of the results of the Wassermann test is difficult and a final assessment depends on the results of both this and other serological tests and the clinical findings. False-positive reactions are sometimes found in leprosy, malaria, sleeping sickness, tuberculosis, infectious mononucleosis and other febrile diseases. Persistent **false-positive** reactions are sometimes found in autoimmune haemolytic anaemia, systemic lupus erythematosus and liver cirrhosis. A commonly performed test is a slide flocculation test using cardiolipin mixed with the patient's serum. This test is preferred by many laboratories because of its simplicity as an alternative to the Wassermann test. It is known as the VDRL (Venereal Diseases Research Laboratory) slide test. When there is doubt a more specific test may have to be employed, e.g. the treponemal immobilisation test, in which motile treponemata can be seen to be immobilised when examined microscopically after exposure to patient's serum. This test is, however, technically complicated and has largely been replaced by an indirect fluorescent antibody (p. 202) test (fluorescent treponemal antibody absorbed, FTA-ABS test). The test is highly specific and sensitive; it is able to detect antibody at all stages of syphilitic infection. The enzyme-linked immunosorbent assay (ELISA) described on page 236 has the potential for large-scale application in syphilis serology.

Complement fixation tests are used widely in the diagnosis of virus diseases. The source of the antigen is usually the infected tissues of animals, or eggs, or infected tissue cultures. The virus is usually extracted from the tissues or cells by differential centrifugation or sometimes by purifying the virus by adsorbing it on to red cells and then eluting it later.

Haemagglutination-inhibition tests
Another useful procedure for the diagnosis of some types of virus

disease is the **haemagglutination-inhibition** test. This depends on the fact that certain viruses, e.g. those of influenza, mumps and parainfluenza, will agglutinate chicken, human and guinea-pig red cells (Fig. 10.8). Other viruses, e.g. the adenoviruses, agglutinate rat or monkey red cells; the reoviruses and many enteroviruses agglutinate human red cells. The test is performed by mixing the virus with the appropriate red cells in the presence of patient's serum. If antibodies to the virus are present the virus will be unable to bring about haemagglutination. These tests are very valuable because of their extreme specificity and their ability to distinguish antibodies to various substrains and variants of viruses, e.g. the influenza virus. The complement fixation test on the other hand is less valuable for detecting these fine differences.

LABORATORY INVESTIGATIONS IN CLINICAL IMMUNOLOGY

Increasing attention is now being paid in the clinical laboratory to the investigation of the role of immune reactions in the **pathogenesis** of disease and to methods of assessing the **functional status** of the immune system in situations where apparent immune dysfunction exists.

Many of the disease states in which immune reactions are believed to be involved in disease pathogenesis have been considered briefly in preceding sections on hypersensitivity reactions and autoimmune states. Immune deficiency states are refered to in Chapter 9. This text is not to be intended to replace the many excellent textbooks dealing with the laboratory aspects of clinical immunology but to provide a simple outline of the main principles of this complex and difficult subject.

Investigation of hypersensitivity states

Antibodies in anaphylactic states
Hay fever and asthma sufferers characteristically have IgE antibodies in their blood. In 1921 Prausnitz and Küstner described a method for the detection of such 'reaginic' antibody performed by injecting a small quantity of serum from the hay fever patient into the skin of a normal subject. The IgE antibody fixes to the cells of the recipient close to the site of injection and when the antigen (or allergen) to which the patient is sensitive (e.g. a pollen extract) is injected at the site, an inflammatory response takes place due to the release of histamine from mast cells (see p. 184). The same type of

reaction can be elicited in the patient by introducing a small quantity of dilute antigen into the skin (Prick test).

IgE antibodies can be quantitated by the radial immunodiffusion technique described on page 226. IgE directed at particular antigens can be assayed by coupling antigen to an insoluble material and mixing the complex with the patient's serum containing IgE antibody against the antigen. After allowing the binding of the IgE antibodies with antigen to take place, unbound serum proteins are washed away and the bound IgE antibody is detected with radio-labelled (^{125}I) anti-IgE antiserum.

Another procedure that can be used to detect sensitization to a particular antigen is to collect peripheral blood leucocytes from the patient and mix them with antigen. The lymphocytes will bind the antigen by their cell membrane receptors, as described on page 47, and the cells will be stimulated to transform in the way described on page 91. Macrophage migration inhibition tests have also been applied on detect sensitisation to antigens. This procedure is described on page 245.

Another laboratory procedure as yet little-used in clinical practice is the determination of the histocompatibility antigen type (p. 161) of the peripheral blood leucocytes. In studies in the United States an association has been found between the occurrence of allergy to ragweed antigen (antigen E) and HLA haplotypes. These studies have been confined so far to a small number of families. The association has been found to occur within particular families, making it possible to identify within a particular family the members at risk and likely to develop the particular ragweed allergy. If these studies are confirmed leucocyte typing may become a useful laboratory aid to the clinician.

Antibodies to inhaled organic material

A condition called 'extrinsic alveolitis' has been recognised in persons who inhale organic material such as fungal spores, dust from various birds or dust from mouldy hay or barley. The lung changes appear to be associated with IgG antibodies formed against the inhaled material and these antibodies are detected by gel diffusion precipitin tests, as described on page 224.

Pulmonary aspergillosis due to inhalation of spores of *Aspergillus fumigatus* sometimes develops in patients with asthma or with an old healed tuberculous cavity, and precipitating antibodies can be detected in their serum. *Candida albicans* respiratory infections can also result in similar antibodies.

Inhalation of *Micromonospora faeni* from mouldy hay can result in a form of alveolitis known as farmer's lung disease, and mouldy barley containing *Aspergillus clavatus* can result in maltworker's lung disease. Gel diffusion tests for precipitating antibodies against antigenic extracts of the microorganisms have proved useful in the diagnosis of the conditions (see also p. 136).

Inhalation of antigens from birds is responsible for bird fancier's lung disease, and here again precipitating IgG antibodies can be detected against avian antigens. The antigens are present in bird serum, feathers and droppings and for the most reliable results material should be used from the particular species of bird to which the patient has been exposed — chickens, pigeons, budgerigars, parrots, and so on.

Antibodies against self-constitutents (autoantibodies)

Organ- (or tissue) specific autoantibodies
Autoantibodies against organ-specific antigens or non-organ-specific antigens are found in a wide range of disease states, as described in Chapter 9. Whilst their role, if any, in the disease process itself is not clear, their presence can be a useful guide as an aid in clinical diagnosis.

Amongst the more common organ-specific autoantibodies are those found in autoimmune haemolytic anaemia. Two main types of antibody have been found: (1) So-called 'warm antibodies' that combine at body temperature with red cells. These are usually of IgG class in contrast to IgM anti-red cell autoantibodies responsible for 'cold antibody' haemolytic anaemia that can be shown to agglutinate red cells at 4°C. The detection of these antibodies usually depends on the use of the Coombs antiglobulin test described on page 230. (2) Leucocyte and platelet autoantibodies have also been described in some rare disease states and are occasionally induced by drugs that combine with these blood components (p. 188).

Organ-specific autoantibodies have been described in the serum of patients with thyroiditis, adrenal disease, pernicious anaemia and disease of the salivary glands (Sjögren's syndrome). The main test here is the fluorescent antibody method (p. 233) with tissue sections of the appropriate tissue; but passive haemagglutination (p. 227) or gel diffusion tests are sometimes used in which red cells are coated with the tissue antigen or the antigen is placed in the wells for the immunodiffusion test (p. 224) with the patient's serum in opposite wells.

Non-organ-specific antibodies

In certain disease states such as rheumatoid arthritis and systemic lupus erythematosus (discussed in Ch. 5) autoantibodies are found in widely distributed antigens not restricted to any one organ or tissue. Autoantibodies in this category are also found in various forms of chronic liver disease.

An agglutination test is widely used for the diagnosis of rheumatoid arthritis; the sera of 70 to 80% of patients with this disease contain an IgM antibody which is able to combine with the IgG globulin from various species. Detection of the antibody depends on the agglutination of sheep red cells or inert particles (polystyrene latex) coated with IgG globulin. Sheep red cells, for example, may be coated with specific rabbit antibody and will then be agglutinated by the IgM antibody in the rheumatoid patient's serum. The antibody s known as **rheumatoid factor**. Occasional low titres (less than 16) are found in normal sera (2 to 5%) and the test is not entirely specific for rheumatoid arthritis.

The fluorescent antibody test is the most commonly used method for the detection of the **antinuclear factor** (ANF) found in the majority of cases of systemic lupus erythematosus. Sections of tissue, e.g. rat liver, are used as the substrate and are layered with patient's serum. Binding of ANF to the liver cell nuclei is detected with fluorescein-labelled antihuman immunoglobulin (see p. 233).

In a liver disease known as primary biliary cirrhosis most patients have antibodies against mitochondrial antigens. These are detected by the fluorescent antibody test with unfixed tissue sections or sometimes by complement fixation tests with rat liver mitochondria. In chronic active hepatitis, and transiently in just over half of patients with infective hepatitis, antibodies are found against smooth muscle actomyosin. The fluorescent antibody test is the method of choice using unfixed sections of rat stomach.

Immune deficiency states

The clinical and immunological aspects of these states are discussed in Chapter 9 and can be seen to involve one or more of the different components of the immune system: (1) the cells responsible for making circulating immunoglobulins, (2) the cells concerned with the cell mediated immune response and (3) the bone marrow stem cells. A wide range of laboratory tests are available to investigate the various forms of deficiency.

Immunoglobulin production. Assay of circulating immunoglobulins can be assessed qualitatively by electrophoresis and quantitatively by immunodiffusion tests. These latter tests are capable of identifying deficiencies of particular classes of immunoglobulin, as described on page 226.

The ability of the patient to make specific immunoglobulin can be tested by **active immunisation** with, for example, a bacterial antigen such as tetanus toxoid and the antibody response measured by a tube precipitation test (p. 222).

The presence of the cells involved in the humoral immune response can be assayed by making use of the fact that the particular cells concerned — the B lymphocytes — have receptors on their surface for the Fc component of the Ig molecule and for the C3 complement component. In the test, sheep red blood cells coated with anti-sheep red cell antibody and complement (in non-lytic quantities) are mixed with peripheral blood leucocytes. The sheep red cells become attached to B lymphocytes by means of the Fc and C3 receptors (that combine ith the antibody and complement on the red cell) forming 'rosettes' (p. 58). The proportion of leucocytes forming such rosettes gives an estimate of the number of B lymphocytes and is normally about 25% of the lymphocytes in human peripheral blood.

Tests of the function of the cell-mediated immune system

Skin tests. The classical method for testing the responsiveness of the cells involved in cell-mediated immunity is the **delayed hypersensitivity skin test** described on page 92. The tuberculin response is the best known example. It is induced by the intradermal injection of 0.1 ml of a 1:1000 dilution (or a greater dilution in a highly sensitive individual) of a protein extract of tubercle bacilli (purified protein derivative, PPD). The reaction is described on page 92; it is only one of a number of similar tests of delayed hypersensitivity such as that using lepromin (in leprosy) and brucellin (in brucellosis). One of the main uses of tests of this type is to detect sensitisation to the relevant microorganism, as for example prior to the use of the BCG vaccine (p. 140) in the prevention of tuberculosis. Clearly in the presence of a positive tuberculin test immunisation with the vaccine will not be called for. A negative reaction in an adult, particularly in one known to have previously shown a positive test, raises the possibility of a defect of the cell-mediated immune system, which in the adult would be likely to be secondary to some disease state affecting the lymphoid tissues such as Hodgkin's disease, multiple myeloma, leukaemia and lymphosarcoma.

Lymphocyte function tests. The thymus-dependent (T) lymphocyte has been pointed to as the main effector cell in cell-mediated immune reactions (Ch. 4). The presence of the T lymphocyte in the peripheral blood can be detected very much in the same way as B lymphocytes can be detected. Instead of using antibody and complement-coated sheep red blood cells as is required for B cells, sheep cells alone are all that is required. T lymphocytes have receptors for sheep erythrocytes and can thus form rosettes when the two types of cell are mixed together. Between 40 and 60% of the human peripheral blood lymphocytes can form rosettes of this type.

Lymphocyte transformation. A particularly useful and widely used assay of lymphocyte function is the lymphocyte transformation test. This is usually carried out using plant phytohaemagglutinin (PHA) as the stimulating agent; the process is described in some detail on p. 92. In other situations a transformation test may be performed with specific antigens to which the individual is believed to be sensitised (e.g. tuberculin). In contrast to the use of PHA, which stimulates a high proportion of T lymphocytes, specific antigen will only stimulate those lymphocytes that are specifically 'committed' to the antigen in question and this is usually only a small portion of the total T lymphocytes. A low level of lymphocyte transformation (when compared with control subjects), either with PHA or specific antigen, indicates impaired cell-mediated immunity (or perhaps absence of previous exposure to the antigen used), whilst increased transformation in the presence of a specific antigen may occur in certain hypersensitivity states, e.g. drug allegies (p. 194).

Migration inhibition. A modification of the macrophage migration inhibition test (see p. 93) using human peripheral blood leucocytes (instead of guinea-pig peritoneal macrophages) can be used in the assessment of cell-mediated immunity. Peripheral blood leucocytes are collected in a small capillary tube in the same way as described in the macrophage inhibition test and, when put in a culture chamber, grow out of the end of the tube in a fan shape. If, however, antigen, to which the cell donor has previously be sensitised, is put into the chamber the leucocytes fail to grow out of the tube. This inhibitory effect is believed to be due to a 'lymphokine' produced by the sensitised lymphocytes on exposure to antigen. This form of assessment of lymphocyte function has very much the same value as the transformation tests referred to above.

Tests of phagocytic cell activity. Defective phagocytic mechanisms are discussed in Chapter 9 and can be assayed in a variety of ways in the laboratory:

1. The ability of phagocytes to respond to a chemotactic agent

(e.g. antigen-antibody complexes in fresh serum) can be measured by inducing the phagocytes to migrate from a chamber through a millipore membrane towards an outer chamber containing the Ag–Ab complexes and serum. The number of phagocytes that respond can be estimated by removing the membrane, staining it with a suitable stain and, under the microscope, counting the number of cells either in the process of passing through the membrane or on the outer side of the membrane.

2. The ability of phagocytes to ingest and kill microorganisms (e.g. staphylococci) or ingest inert particles such as latex or oil droplets can be determined by microscopic examination of cell preparations mixed with the microorganism or inert particle. Killing of microorganisms within phagocytes can be estimated by disrupting the cells (e.g. by distilled water) and counting the colonies of microorganisms that can be grown on a suitable nutrient agar plate.

3. The normal functioning of phagocyte lysosomal enzyme activity can be assessed by a dye reduction test using tetrazolium nitroblue. A defect on the part of the patient's cells can be detected by a failure of the leucocytes to reoxidise the reduced colourless dye to its blue colour. A deficiency of this function is characteristic of chronic granulomatous disease (p. 196).

The complement system. Changes in the levels of this complex group of serum protein constituents (see Ch. 2) are often a reflection of an underlying disease process. **Raised** levels of the components are frequently found in acute inflammatory and infective disease states in conjunction with raised levels of 'acute phase proteins' such as C reactive protein.

Reduction in complement levels is a more useful guide to the understanding of disease pathogenesis and fall into two categories: (1) primary deficiencies — genetically determined deficiencies of complement components, and (2) secondary deficiencies — as a consequence of complement consuming antibody-antigen interactions or associated with renal or liver disease.

The genetically determined deficiencies are rare conditions, the best known of which is the deficiency of C1 esterase inhibitor (see p. 196). Very rare deficiencies of other components (C3, C1, C5) have been described.

The secondary deficiencies are much more frequently found and most often occur in renal disease such as post-streptococcal nephritis, in the nephritis of systemic lupus erythematosis and in chronic membrano-proliferative glomerulonephritis. Low levels also occur in serum sickness (immune complex disease), bacterial septicaemia, malaria and in various forms of liver disease.

In the laboratory two main types of assay are available: (1) functional tests of the haemolytic activity of the complement system, and (2) immunochemical estimation of the levels of individual complement components.

Haemolytic activity of the complement system is usually assayed by the method described by Mayer, which measures the number of 'units' of complement per ml of serum. A unit of complement is defined as the quality required to lyse 50% of a standard sheep cell suspension, optimally sensitised with anti-sheep cell antibody. The volume, buffer components and incubation conditions are likewise defined. The test is sometimes referred to as a CH50 assay.

Estimation of individual components, whilst possible by assays of their functional activity, is usually performed by immunochemical methods utilising specific antisera against individual components. The method of choice is the quantitative radial immunodiffusion test (p. 227) in which the antisera are incorporated in the agar and the serum specimens are placed in the wells. Commercially prepared plates are available for a wide range of complement components.

Immune complex detection. In the circulation the potentially pathogenic complexes are those found in antigen excess. There is now convincing evidence that they play a role in the pathogenesis of rheumatoid arthritis, glomerulonephritis, polyarteritis, rheumatic fever and a number of infective states discussed in Chapter 5 (p. 190). In most instances, complement activation seems likely to be responsible for the inflammatory changes that occur, with chemotaxis of neutrophils and release of lysosomal enzymes as the prime factors involved (see Ch. 2, p. 20).

The following detection methods in general require specialised laboratory facilities: (a) electron-microscopic demonstration of complexes in tissues, such as those found in the liver of patients with hepatitis B virus infections; (b) precipitation of complexes in the cold, cryoprecipitation, and subsequent identification of microbial antigens e.g., hepatitis B antigens; (c) detection of bound complement components (e.g. C1q) in the complexes, often after precipitation by polyethylene glycol. The principle of the assay is that the naturally bound C1q is removed with Na_2EDTA, a radiolabelled C1q is then added, followed by polyethylene glycol to precipitate the complexes. The C1q remaining in the supernatant is then measured, allowing the estimation of the bound C1q; (d) immunobiological tests such as aggregation of platelets and inhibition of antibody-mediated cytotoxicity. The latter test is quite widely used and involves inhibition of the killing by non-sensitised lymphocytes of target cells (e.g. Chang cells, a line of human liver cells) coated with antibody. If immune complexes are added to the lymphocytes, their Fc receptors are blocked by the antibody in the complexes so that the receptors cannot bind the antibody on the target cell.

Other tests

A number of miscellaneous clinical immunological investigations are sometimes called for and include examination of biopsy material for deposits of antibody or complement by immunofluorescence, estimation of cryoglobulins, radioimmunoassay for the presence of hepatitis B antigen and characterisation of monoclonal antibodies by immunoelectrophoresis or examination of bone marrow by immunofluorescence. In diagnosis of virus infection speed is important, enabling public health control measures to be started and more immediate care for the patient.

The ELISA assay has been discussed and is likely to have wide applications. Assay of specific IgM may be helpful in atypical measles or mumps and in certain arbovirus infections. Electron microscopic examination is widely used for biopsy material as well as the fluorescent antibody technique.

Most of these procedures require specialised laboratory facilities not generally available in the routine clinical pathology laboratory.

FURTHER READING

Campbell D H, Garvey J S, Cremer N E, Sussdorf D 1963 Methods in immunology. Benjamin, New York
Duguid J P, Marmion B P, Swain R H A 1978 Mackie and McCartney medical microbiology, a guide to the laboratory diagnosis and control of infection, 13th edn. Churchill Livingstone, Edinburgh
Glynn L E, Reading C A 1981 Immunological investigation of connective tissue diseases. Churchill Livingstone, Edinburgh
Hudson L, Hay F C 1980 Practical immunology, 2nd edn. Blackwell, Oxford
Nairn R C 1969 Fluorescent protein tracing, 3rd edn. Churchill Livingstone, Edinburgh
Nowotny A 1969 Basic exercises in immunochemistry. Springer, Berlin
Thompson R A 1974 The practice of clinical immunology. Arnold, London
Thompson R A (ed) 1981 Techniques in clinical immunology, 2nd edn. Blackwell, Oxford
Weir D M, Herzenberg L 1983 Handbook of experimental immunology, 4th edn. Blackwell, Oxford
Wilkinson A E 1970 The positive Wassermann reaction; investigation and interpretation. British Journal of Hospital Medicine 4: 47
Williams C A, Chase M W 1968 Methods in immunology and immunochemistry. Academic Press, New York
World Health Organisation 1981 Technical report series no. 661: Rapid laboratory techniques for the diagnosis of viral infections. WHO, Geneva

Index

Page numbers in **bold** indicate the location of the main discussion of a subject.

250 INDEX